Keep ✓

S0-BFO-655

Bradley, Denise J.

RC
660
.B73
1987
c 2

What does it feel
like to have
diabetes?

OCT 1 2 1993	DATE DUE	
NOV 3 0 1993 MAY 2 3 1996		
APR 2 6 1994 MAY 2 2 1997		
MAY 1994		
DEC 0 6 1994		
DEC 1 8 1994		
MAR 2 8 1995		
APR 1 1 1995		
MAY 0 9 1995		
MAY 2 3 1995		
FEB 2 7 1996		

WHAT DOES IT FEEL LIKE
TO HAVE DIABETES?

WHAT DOES IT FEEL LIKE TO HAVE DIABETES?

A Diary of Events in the Life of a Diabetic

By

DENISE J. BRADLEY

With Forewords by

Martin J. Conway, M.D.

and

Kathryn Hazard, R.N., M.S.N.

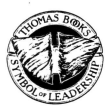

CHARLES C THOMAS • PUBLISHER
Springfield • Illinois • U.S.A.

6/93
RC
660
.B73
1987
C 2

Published and Distributed Throughout the World by
CHARLES C THOMAS • PUBLISHER
2600 South First Street
Springfield, Illinois 62794-9265

This book is protected by copyright. No part of
it may be reproduced in any manner without
written permission from the publisher.

© *1987 by* CHARLES C THOMAS • PUBLISHER
ISBN 0-398-05367-7
Library of Congress Catalog Card Number: 87-11217

With THOMAS BOOKS *careful attention is given to all details of manufacturing and design. It is the Publisher's desire to present books that are satisfactory as to their physical qualities and artistic possibilities and appropriate for their particular use.* THOMAS BOOKS *will be true to those laws of quality that assure a good name and good will.*

Printed in the United States of America
Q-R-3

Library of Congress Cataloging in Publication Data
Bradley, Denise J.
    What does it feel like to have diabetes?

    1. Bradley, Denise J. — Health. 2. Diabetics —
United States — Biography. 3. Diabetes — Psycho-
logical aspects. I. Title [DNLM: 1. Diabetes
Mellitus — personal narratives. 2. Diabetes Melli-
tus — popular works.   WK 850 B811w]
RC660.B73 1987   362.1'96462 [B]   87-11217
ISBN 0-398-05367-7

To Steve
your love and wit light up my life

To Mother
your enthusiasm is forever inspiring

To both of you
thank you for believing in me and this book

FOREWORD

THIS WORK represents the events which may occur in the life of a diabetic, beginning with the onset of diabetes and proceeding to the level of acceptance in dealing with the process in a realistic fashion. From a physician's standpoint, I believe that Denise Bradley has identified a number of the basic problems of living which the diabetic may go through, beginning with the early part of learning how to get around some of the restrictions that the initial diagnosis imposes. This period of denial, ignorance and finally coming to grips with the individual responsibility in managing the problem is well documented in this book and highlights for the diabetic the very real and human difficulties to be faced in dealing with the disease.

There is provided herein for the individual with diabetes a totally different dimension of the disease than is available in the usual materials that are given to him or to her to read, and which deal in a large part with diabetes as seen through the eyes of the physician. Such books as are normally provided for the diabetic give much in the way of worthwhile facts but provide virtually no insight into the psychological and living difficulties the diabetic must face to effectively accommodate, and finally establish a symbiotic relationship — if the diabetic is going to function at all effectively — with day-to-day living.

In contrast to many other books presented by diabetics, this one is not cluttered with the usual type of physiology, discussions of how to, and so on. It is rather a documentary trip of the personal experiences of the author in working with the diagnosis of diabetes mellitus and its complications.

I feel strongly that the book highlights a number of important areas that neither physicians nor other health care providers have much insight into and, consequently, are not very effectively addressed in most of the published material related to diabetes and its difficulties.

The book makes excellent reading and is an important information base relative to the behavioral and psychologic problems the diabetic must face. It is written almost as an autobiography, providing exclusive insight into these difficult areas which are so often ineffectively addressed in so much of the materials which are presented to patients and their families.

I support this book as being very useful not only to the diabetic population but also to the multiplicity of health care providers who deal on a regular basis with diabetes.

Martin J. Conway, M.D.
Head, Section of Endocrinology
Lovelace Medical Center
Albuquerque, New Mexico

FOREWORD

DIABETES is a challenging, chronic illness to master. The impact of diabetes plays not only on the individual's physical being but also on his/her emotional, economic and interpersonal health. Unlike such temporary illnesses as appendicitis or the flu, diabetes is unrelentingly permanent. A lifetime of vigilance is required in every facet of living along with a sound knowledge base of disease management, significant resources, and multiple coping skills. With few conditions do today's successes so greatly determine one's future health and well being.

Because of the complexity of diabetes, many health care professionals, as well as people living with diabetes, have only a rudimentary comprehension of disease management. This book provides valuable insight for all touched by diabetes. The reality of living with diabetes through the life cycles, and the struggles of coping with a traumatic life event, are vividly chronicled. As the health care professional, or person living with diabetes, follows Denise Bradley as she eventually triumphs over diabetes, they will gain a deeper understanding of their own venture efforts to conquer this major obstacle to health and happiness.

Kathryn Hazard, R.N., M.S., C.D.E.
Diabetes Nurse Specialist
Southwest Community Health
Services Affiliates
Albuquerque, New Mexico

INTRODUCTION

WHAT DOES it feel like to have diabetes? To take shots? To have insulin reactions? To have others be watchdogs of your eating behavior? To slowly lose your vision? How can diabetes be considered an opportunity rather than a misfortune? Whether you are a diabetic yourself, the parent of a diabetic, a friend, coworker, or doctor to a diabetic, this book has been written to help give you an emotional understanding of diabetes.

The diabetic experience has many facets beyond the physical disease process and what lack of insulin does to the body.

First and foremost is the mental stress on the diabetic, stemming both from the unstable nature of the disease, and from the huge responsibility placed on him, in which his very behavior on a day-to-day basis determines his present, as well as his future, health and well-being. There is also the strain on family interactions, psychological and financial, which living with diabetes can bring.

There is the diabetic's relationship to food and eating, and the recurring battles against temptation and guilt. There are the ever-present fears of possible health complications, compounded by the fact that deterioration begins with imperceptible changes in the body. There are the myths and misconceptions about diabetes, perpetuated by society and the medical community, which constantly confront the diabetic. And, because the diabetic often feels like he is on trial to defend his performance as a "good diabetic," there is frequently a lack of communication between him and his doctor.

It is inevitable that at some time in your life as a diabetic, or in your involvement with a diabetic, any or all of these problems will arise. This book is a place for you to turn to, not only for answers, but for understanding.

I present here a personal account of some of my experiences as a diabetic, and an exploration of the "feeling" side of diabetes. By sharing my story and what the effects of my diabetes were on myself and my family, I hope to spare you some of the frustrations and complications of the disease, and to impart some of the positive aspects which are possible. Hopefully, you will learn both from our mistakes and our successes. This book will teach only by showing and not by telling.

I developed diabetes when I was 11 years old. Before the diagnosis was made, I lost 40 pounds and lapsed into a coma. From that point on my life was changed. The excitement of something new in my life wore off quickly, and I was faced with the daily challenges of diabetes. Over the next many years I underwent the range of extremes of living with a chronic disease: denial, addiction, and loss of self-esteem. I was overwhelmed by guilty feelings I could not understand, and instead of controlling my diabetes, I let the diabetes control me.

Although my family loved me and tried to help, our relationships were strained. We were not consciously aware of the impact diabetes had on us as a family, or that what I needed most was emotional support.

Nearly 20 years went by before I came to see diabetes as a strength to build on rather than a weakness to fall back on. The change in my attitude and behavior did not happen overnight. But, the important thing is that despite the long-term abuse and damage to my body, I was still able to turn my health almost totally around. Here I will take you through that learning process with candor, empathy, and humor. It is my endeavor that through these pages you will be empowered with a good feeling about diabetes, and a strong sense of the control you can have over your own health and life.

Denise J. Bradley

CONTENTS

     Onset of diabetes at age 11
     Illness brings positive attention
     Symptoms/Warning signs of diabetes
     Limited comprehension of disease and its impact

     Birth of twins is big news
     The subject of twins
     My childhood as a twin
     Diabetes is catalyst for change in twin relationship

     First time to "cheat" on diet
     Feeling unique/Feeling outcast
     Learning to give insulin injections
     Insulin reactions: what they are and how they feel

     First schoolyear with diabetes/Attitudes of friends
     Doctor's failure to communicate
     Overeating causes family friction
     Bizarre incident frightens my family

WHAT DOES IT FEEL LIKE
TO HAVE DIABETES?

Chapter One

WAKING UP TO A NEW LIFE

I KNEW SOMETHING was wrong the instant I opened my eyes. As when awakening from a nightmare, my body was rigid with fright and I did not know if I could not or dare not, move. Without turning my head or eyes, I attempted to focus on what was in my direct line of vision. Whatever I was looking at was not only unfamiliar, but completely incomprehensible, and that scared me. I closed my eyes and prayed silently that I was dreaming.

After a few moments, I cautiously peeked out from behind my eyelashes. Seeing again the strange sight perpetuated my fear and made me angry, too. I did not want to be awake and acknowledge that what I was looking at was real, for if it was real, then sooner or later I would have to face it. "Face what?" I thought, as my mind strained for an explanation.

If I were just waking up, I should be looking at my bedroom ceiling . . . that was it! I was looking at a ceiling, but it was not my ceiling. Instead of cheery sunlight on pastel print, there was a glaring metal object which I resented being there.

By this time even though I had not moved a muscle, I could tell that I was lying flat on my back with my arms stretched out along the sides of my body. I thought if I could just touch my face or my chest, I would be able to make some sense out of all this. Gathering courage, I tried lifting one of my arms, but it would not move. A sick sensation filled my stomach. Now I wanted desperately to move, but felt pinned down by some outer force. I turned my head a fraction of an inch to the left and saw more stark metal along the length of what I had to assume was a bed. This sight was too much for me. My emotions overtook my tension and I cried out.

"Denny, are you all right?"

What a relief to hear my father's voice. At once he was by my side, his warm hands touching me as he gently kissed my cheek.

"Everything is okay, darlin'. I'm here," he said. "You're in the hospital. You got sick and we had to bring you here. The bars are to keep you from falling out of bed."

I looked down at my arms, puzzled. Daddy picked up on my fear and confusion. He explained that my arms were taped to boards and the boards were taped to the bed. This was because there were needles in my veins and if I moved the wrong way, they might come out. I raised my head to look around and all I saw was white—the blankets, the sheets, my nightgown, and my arms which were encased in white tape from the mid-biceps to the wrists. It was impossible to move my arms with all that tape. I felt weak and sleepy as I laid my head back on the pillow. I had had enough explanations for the time being, and feeling somewhat comforted, I slept.

I awoke a short time later and was at once aware of being extremely cold, especially in my arms. I glanced at my hands and noticed that my wrists were puffed up the size of golf balls. I called out to my father that I was freezing and that my wrists looked funny. He assured me that the nurses were keeping a close watch on me. Daddy admitted not knowing what caused the puffiness, but he said he would ask the nurse about it the next time she came into my room.

The news that I was awake apparently traveled quickly. Soon various white-jacketed people were streaming in and out of my room. They all seemed happy that I was awake and kept asking me how I felt. I answered each by repeating that my arms were very cold, but that I felt pretty good.

Finally, a nurse told me that the cold and puffiness were normal reactions to having needles in my veins and that the discomfort would go away. She tucked heated, dry towels around my arms and I was grateful for the warmth.

My attention was soon diverted from my body by the bustling activity going on around me. Everyone was friendly and always explained who they were and what they were going to do to me. One nurse kept putting a thermometer in my mouth, another took my blood pressure every few minutes, and still another kept taking blood from my arm and giving me shots.

I was still weak and just allowed all this to go on around me without raising any objections. It was all new and fascinating to me as an 11-year-old girl who had never been in the hospital before. I could not remember ever getting quite this much attention.

Had I been alone in this situation, things may not have gone so smoothly. My father's presence made all the difference. He remained close at hand and even spent the nights in a big stuffed chair that had been brought in and placed next to my bed. I felt so loved and secure and lucky to have him there. Even though I still did not know what was wrong with me, everything would be all right because he said it would be.

The busy bedside routine continued the next morning, but with an additional surprise. A nurse walked in carrying a ceramic vase of colorful flowers and said they were for me. I was truly amazed! To my delight, the rest of that day and for several days to follow, more flowers, cards, and gifts poured in. My get well wishes included seven pairs of pajamas, two robes, plants, comic books, games, and numerous phone calls and visitors. I had never been given flowers or plants and was accustomed to receiving cards and gifts only at Christmas and on my birthday. All of this just because I was sick . . .

I was a bit disappointed that my father could not stay with me all the time, but I was never left alone. While Daddy was at work, my stepmother Janet filled in for him. She played games with me and we joked with the nurses. I was glad for her company. Since I was on the children's floor, Janet and I would walk around and visit some of the other kids. One baby boy was wrapped in bandages so that only his face was showing. We found out that his babysitter had accidently dropped hot coffee on him. This upset me and I made it a point to check regularly with the nurses about his progress.

One morning a nurse came into my room accompanied by a round-faced, friendly looking man and introduced him as my doctor. He had red hair and freckles and I always remembered who he was. He laughed a lot and was very nice to me and I enjoyed his visits to my room. He said he was happy to see me looking so well as I had been quite a sick little girl when I was brought in.

Each day I could feel myself getting stronger and more alert. One evening Daddy told me that even though I was getting better and feeling good, I had a disease that would not go away. This disease was the reason I had been so sick. The disease was called diabetes. I would have to remain in the hospital another week-and-a-half to learn how to take care of myself. Daddy said we would learn together.

I took this news rather nonchalantly. I tried pronouncing the name "di-a-bee-tis" a few times and remarked that it sounded funny. My limited concept of the word *dis*ease had come from television and movies.

Disease to me was something like cancer where a person went to the hospital and later died or had an operation and got well. Or, disease could be where a person was crippled and wound up in a wheelchair or had therapy to learn to walk again.

However, none of these situations applied to me. I could walk and talk. I still retained my arms and legs, and, most importantly, I felt great. This diabetes couldn't be too bad if I felt this good.

The next day I called my mother to tell her what had happened. Of course, Daddy had called her as soon as I went into the hospital. I felt strange telling her I had a disease. Even to me it seemed like a story that had been made up. It didn't mean anything to me. But, my mother and grandma were more anxious about the disease than I was and kept asking me if I was okay. I sounded so bright and cheerful on the phone that I calmed their immediate fears. Later, Mother told me she was making plans to drive to Kansas City to see me. Since I felt fine, I didn't know why she would drive all the way from New Mexico, but I knew she loved me very much and I guess she needed to see for herself.

Because Janet stayed with me during the day, that left my twin sister Deb at home alone with April, our three-year-old half sister. Deb called me daily to report on news from the outside world and I, in turn, shared what was happening to me. She told me that I had missed seeing the ambulance that took me to the hospital. I was a little jealous when she said that the siren had been blaring. She explained that I was put on a stretcher and that Janet rode along in the ambulance. It had been scary because none of them knew what was wrong with me.

Deb's phone calls got me to thinking about the events that led up to me being in the hospital. My twin and I had just graduated from fifth grade with a whole summer ahead of us. Ordinarily I was a typical, active child riding my bike, playing games, and forever thinking up ways to fill the endless days of vacation.

But this June had started out differently. I had been so tired. Having minimal energy, I frequently wanted to lie down and rest, just for a minute. I was also more thirsty than usual and could hardly wait until the ice cream truck drove by, its bell signaling that I could buy a cold, wet popsicle. I found myself day-dreaming about popsicles and of drinking all the liquid I could get my hands on.

Watching Deb and our friends run around invoked little interest in me to join them. Food was not of much interest either. All I cared about was getting enough to drink. What my family and I had no way of knowing was that I was actually dehydrating very, very slowly.

About the middle of June Deb and I began packing for our annual two-week trip to visit our father. This was always a time of great anticipation for us, as we were close to our father and loved him very much. Having spent so little time together since our parents' divorce when we were three years old, our visits with Daddy were extra special.

This summer I wanted to go to Kansas City even though the thought of a long train trip seemed tiring. I compensated for this by thinking that as soon as the traveling was over, I could rest all I wanted at Daddy's house. I did not let my apprehensions be known to my family, however, fearing they may inquire about my health and postpone or cancel the trip. As the day of departure neared, Mother told me that I looked a little pale and wanted to know how I was feeling. I confided that I had a slight stomachache, but added that it was probably just the flu. I promised to have Daddy take me to the doctor if I got worse. She hesitated but did not push the issue because she knew how much the trip meant to me.

As it turned out, Mother was right to have had her doubts. She regretted later about having let me go, but at the time she acted out of a desire to see me happy. Just before Deb and I were ready to get on the train, I could tell that Mother was upset. She considered calling off the trip, but Deb came to my rescue and said she would watch me and also tell Daddy about Mother's concerns. Deb's argument along with my persistence persuaded Mother, and we climbed aboard.

My sister and I had been riding the train to Kansas City by ourselves since we were eight years old and we truly loved it. Of course, riding without an adult added to the excitement and made us feel grown up. The train we took was the old Santa Fe Chief. Going by train in those days was an adventure, expecially for children. There were always several children traveling alone and the conductors and porters protectively took us under their wings. They were empathetic to our fears and our excitement. While answering all our questions, they saw to it that we had everything we might need, including pillows which rented for 25 cents.

It's difficult to say what Deb and I liked best about the train, whether it was visiting the snack counter to buy Cheese Nips® and comic books, or bravely crossing from one car to another, or having meals in the dining car. We liked to watch the black waiters in their white uniforms expertly balancing trays of food, seemingly unaware of the jostling back-and-forth of the cars. For dessert we liked to order vanilla ice cream because we thought it looked like fresh cakes of Ivory® soap.

One year we both received Chatty Cathy® talking dolls for Christmas and took them on the train with us. The waiters joked with us and asked our dolls what they would like to order. We got a kick out of that!

It was customary to arrive in Kansas City before dawn. The conductors would come around to the passengers who would be departing and quietly whisper that the next stop was Kansas City. At this time of day, the only illumination came from tiny footlights along the aisle. All of us kids thought it was fun to run around in the dark while everyone else was sleeping. The conductors would hang out the open doors as we slowed to a stop. When one would yell "Kansas City!", I'd get butterflies in my stomach.

As soon as the train stopped, we would look out the window and spot our father standing on the platform. We couldn't get out fast enough. For the next few moments it was hugs and kisses galore. We were always openly affectionate with one another. This time, after our initial greeting, Daddy inquired about our health. I told him about my stomachache and thirst and we hurried to get home.

The first few days of our visit were not pleasant for me. Deb, April, and I spent most of our time in April's plastic swimming pool which had been set up in their huge, grassy backyard. I would lie in the pool for hours, wishing I could absorb all that water into me. Quietly and motionless I lay there, mumbling "yes" to Deb's repeated question, "Denise, are you okay?" Deb later told me that my stillness had frightened her.

My stomachache turned into a sideache and I felt more weak than ever. I stayed in bed, ate little, and kept asking for water. Daddy called the doctor and between them they decided I had the flu. I also vomited some, which made the diagnosis seem accurate. But, when the sideache grew so severe that I was doubled over in pain, Daddy made a doctor's appointment for the following day. I did not want to go because from Daddy's house to anywhere was a long ride and I didn't think I could sit up that long.

When it came time to leave for the doctor's, Janet and Deb helped me to the car. I sat next to a window in the back of the small gray and white Fiat. Even without Daddy, there was no room to stretch out on the seat. The ride was torturous. When I tried to lean on the door for support, the car's movement kept my head knocking against the window. It seemed like the trip would never end. I wanted to lie down and be very still.

Immediately upon entering the doctor's office, I asked Janet if there was a drinking fountain nearby. She pointed me in the right direction after I declined her offer of assistance in getting there. The fountain was one of the new electric models with ice-cold water and I did not want to stop drinking and letting the refreshing liquid stream over my face.

Standing there, aware of nothing but the heavenly cool water is the last thing I remember. My next conscious moment was the frightening instant when I awoke in the hospital room. Daddy filled in the missing gaps for me. He described how I had collapsed in front of the drinking fountain just as a doctor was walking by. The doctor carried me to an examining table, observed my visible symptoms, and took my vital signs. He also noticed that my breath had a fruity, acrid smell which is a strong indication of diabetes being present. He called for an ambulance at once. The fact that I had no memory of the 24 hours that followed was hard for me to grasp.

One evening when my father walked into my hospital room, he was carrying a book which he said was about diabetes. He was going to read to me from the book every night. I welcomed this because for as long as I could remember, Daddy had read bedtime stories to Deb and me. We'd beg him to read our favorite ones over and over. In time he had memorized two of the stories which were full of nonsensical names and phrases. He put so much animation and inflection into his reading that it was like watching a play. At the time our father was a disc jockey. He has a very pleasing voice and to this day, I can listen to him talk for hours.

As he read to me from the book about my disease, I attempted to comprehend and make sense of it all. Occasionally, I would ask questions. Daddy was never bothered by them and answered in a way that I could understand, or at least I thought I did.

Early in the book, we discovered that the most common warning signs or symptoms of diabetes are incessant thirst, frequent urination, tiredness, lack of energy, and weight loss. All of these had occurred in me. Daddy mentioned that when he first saw me at the train station, he had been shocked at how pale and thin I was, and described me as having looked like a skeleton. But he had said nothing because he did not want to upset Deb or me.

The doctor estimated that I had lost about 40 pounds since the onset of the disease. He told my father I might have died if I had not been brought in for another couple of days.

While my mother did detect a change in me, it is understandable why she did not become alarmed at my weight loss. It is likely that I lost the weight over several weeks and even months. Besides that, I had eaten normally up until the previous two weeks. Adding to the cover-up was the fact that Deb and I were at the lanky stage of development when children look thin anyway. Daddy, however, had not seen me for a year and spotted a difference between Deb and me as soon as we stepped off the train.

When Mother learned of the symptoms, she admitted noticing me drinking a lot and going to the bathroom more often, but had assumed the summer heat was responsible for my behavior.

The book Daddy read to me stressed over and over that a diabetic could lead a normal life. Daddy emphasized these words and it all seemed so simple. Unfortunately, most of the text, which offered prescriptions for this "normal life" meant little to me. It was not difficult understanding the words, but the concepts were just not real to me.

Maybe it was like listening to one of my bedtime stories, something I liked to hear but to be forgotten later. It was special that Daddy was reading a book just for me. The delicious sound of syllables forming words and words forming sentences all made by my father's voice had me in a pleasant state of relaxation and security. Little did I know how long it would take for me to comprehend what I was now hearing.

Daddy explained that I would have to take shots every day and I would be learning to give them to myself. I did not think much about that, but what did disturb me was being told I would have to give up eating sweets. I took this news the hardest of all and thought about it a long time.

At bedtime one night I asked, "Daddy, does this mean I can't go Trick-or-Treating anymore?"

"Yes, baby," he replied.

I turned over in bed so that he could not see the silent tears that began trickling down my cheeks. I felt silly crying over candy, but as I dozed off I resented the unknown thief of one of my youthful joys.

How curious that the prospect of giving myself shots did not phase me, but being told I could not have candy made me feel like my childhood was being taken from me.

Chapter Two

THE BIGGEST HIT OF THE YEAR!

EVERYONE GETS excited at the birth of twins. From the moment Deb and I arrived on the scene, we were a big hit. Of course, being born in a small town (population 4,000) and being the first twins born there in many years didn't hurt any. The name of the town was also unique, Truth or Consequences. It was named after the popular Ralph Edwards game show of the same name.

To announce our arrival, our parents sent out clever birth announcements:

> Radio Station B R A D L E Y
> Broadcasting from Truth or Consequences, New Mexico
> proudly presents the biggest hit of the year:
>
> IT'S IDENTICAL TWINS!!!
>
> Setting: St. Ann's Hospital
> Time: January 8, 1952
>
> Cast of Characters:
> Charlotte Mae Bradley, Mother
> Debra Jean, 2 lbs., 6 oz.
> Denise Jane, 3 lbs., 11½ oz.
>
> Producer: Sam Bradley
> Manager: Dr. H. F. Maloney

Not a bad review! Our father had already gained some notoriety as the sole disc jockey for the town's only radio station KCHS. One of the local newspapers, *The Herald*, ran this brief item the day we were born:

> "Looks like the radio finally got ahead of the newspaper. And Sam Bradley is the boy who did it. On January 8, Sam became the proud papa of twin girls. So if he has that worn out, tired feeling in his voice on the early morning newscast, it could have been he was up all night warming bottles and mixing formulas."

Articles appeared in other papers and bulletins. Our father kept the excitement going by using his radio show to run a contest to "Name the Twins." He and our mother had fun going through the entries, which included some rather strange suggestions. Somehow I cannot picture Deb and I being known as Clidece and Clidell! Ironically, it was our aunt Billy Jean who sent in the winning names Denise and Debra.

The appeal of twins seems to come from the fact that they are out of the ordinary. The sight of twins is intriguing to most people, including other twins. While the frequent identical clothes and hairstyles on twins is enough to elicit stares and comments, the novelty is even greater if the pair acts alike.

People often ask if certain twins are identical, meaning are the twins exactly alike physically. Actually, identical refers only to the fact that the twins came from one egg, not two. They may or may not look exactly alike.

In noticing the similarities and differences between twins, there is often an element of delight in observing how much alike one pair is. When there are no obvious likenesses, people say with regret, "they don't even look alike," as if something went wrong in the production.

Without even trying, twins stand out in a crowd and receive attention from all. Babies and small children are especially noticed because they seem to be little toys created for the purpose of looking and performing alike. Strangers will even approach a parent with twins to remark how much the children look alike or how cute they are. The attraction is the same whether the twins are two boys or two girls. At the age of four, my sister and I had very short hair and could pass for either sex depending on what we were wearing. If we had jeans on, our mother often received compliments about her darling twin boys.

For me, being a twin is unique. Deb and I not only look alike, we also laugh and talk alike, and our mannerisms and facial expressions are so similar that at times we appear to be imitating one another. I will catch myself sounding just like my sister and at that moment I feel like I am her and not myself. It is not unusual for us to have extra sensory communication and accurately sense the other's feelings, even if we happen to be separated by great distances. There are times when I "just had a feeling" that Deb was upset only to call and find out that she was indeed upset and had been planning to call me and talk about it. In various situations, each of us knows exactly what the other's reaction would be if she were in similar circumstances.

I do not recall our infant years as twins. For that there are photograph albums and family movies, which are pictorial accounts of how closely our lives were intertwined. The only way to distinguish us is by my slightly larger size. Pictures of birthdays and Christmas time show us in identical outfits while opening gifts that include the same dolls, the same stuffed toys, and more matching outfits. It was always an either/or situation. Either we received the same gift, or we shared one gift.

At our first birthday party, which was also written up in the paper, we shared a big butterfly cake, created by our grandmother. Each of our names was printed on one wing.

As we grew older, the necessity of giving both of us the same gifts wore off, and we often had to share a single gift from someone. This, however, was not as traumatic as the times we received separate and different gifts. Jealousies were strong. I would make Deb promise to let me play with her toy, and she would make me promise the same.

Another common sight in our family albums are pictures of Deb, me, and one of our friends. Deb and I always stood on either side of our shared friend. We never did have individual friends until high school. I suppose sharing a friend was no different than sharing a toy. It was better than each of us having someone different, and I am sure our friends did not mind getting attention from both of us.

We, of course, were known as a single entity, "the twins." "Can the twins come out and play?" was a question heard constantly around our home. I think others use this collective term so as not to show favoritism of one twin over the other. It was almost as if, since we looked alike, we should be treated alike. Perhaps our friends believed they might be violating an unwritten code if they singled out either of us by asking only Deb or I to play.

Occasionally one of our girlfriends would, in a hushed voice, confess that she liked me better than Deb, or that she thought I was prettier. But, she would always be quick to add, "Don't tell Deb I said that!" as if even I must not differentiate between us. No doubt Deb was approached in the same secretive manner.

Deb and I were extremely close from the very beginning. We thoroughly enjoyed being alike and doing things together, and we wanted to keep it that way. After being in the same class for kindergarten, we assumed we would always be together. Therefore, we were upset when we were told we had to enroll in separate first grade classes. We had heard that twins are sometimes kept together for emotional reasons, and it was our hope that the school officials would find this to be in our best interest too. Apparently a split was considered beneficial for us. We compensated by always being together at recess and lunchtime.

During our early years, Deb and I were equal when it came to our academic performance and athletic abilities. Any rivalry between us was associated more with fun than competition. Halloween was a special event for us. It was the only time during the year when we dressed differently. One of my costumes was "Casper the Friendly Ghost" in contrast to Deb's Wicked Witch outfit. For the two weeks following the big night, Deb and I raced home after school, emptied the contents of our Trick or Treat bags onto the bedroom floor, and took an inventory of what candy we had left. We had the same favorites and divided the candy into ranks. Top ranking went to miniature candy bars, which we liked the best and tried to resist eating until the last. Next came caramels, bubble gum, suckers, and hard candy. Fruit and cookies were boring and didn't count, although popcorn balls did have some standing. It was a challenge to enjoy eating our candy while trying to retain an equal or larger amount of it left over than the other had.

We naturally had our share of childhood arguments and fights, but they were overshadowed by the close bond we had developed. Uncomfortable situations were less frightening and new experiences were doubly exciting because there was always someone to share them with. We believed that we were special and lucky to have been born twins. It was a wonderful way to go through childhood, sharing ups-and-downs with the one person in the world closest to you.

Diabetes changed all that. For the first time in our lives, there was something we could not share, even if we had wanted to. From that time on, our parallel lives began to slowly angle off in different directions as we dealt with the unexpected intruder.

Although unaware of it at the time, perhaps I welcomed the sudden attention and change in my life. Maybe it was a way to be different, a way to stand out, a way to start experiencing myself as "Denise the individual" rather than as "Denise the twin." The wonderful rapport Deb and I knew and enjoyed was soon to be altered. But these impending changes were years away from consciousness as I lay in my hospital bed surrounded by gifts and caring, attentive people.

Chapter Three

LEARNING THE PART

ALTHOUGH many activities continued to swirl around me, I was getting bored after a week-and-a-half in the hospital. The lessons I was learning about my disease were interesting enough to hold my attention for awhile, but I was still a normal child and longed to be outdoors and physically active. I missed my twin intensely and I felt deprived of the vacation time we were supposed to be spending with our father.

I was also tired of the large amounts of food I was given each day, not being used to eating three big meals plus frequent snacks of two-inch thick sandwiches and cartons of milk. I guess they wanted to fatten me up before releasing me, since I had looked so pathetic and undernourished when I was brought in.

During one meal I complained to Janet that I just could not eat everything on my tray. She told me I might get home sooner if I forced myself to eat it all. That was the best argument she could have used. I was inspired to finish every crumb and I began to imagine myself running and playing with Deb and our friends.

The eating apparently paid off, for I was released from the hospital a few days later. I was so excited! My doctor and nurses stopped by my room to say good-bye and to wish me luck. Along with all my presents, I packed the numerous personal items which all hospital patients accumulate, knowing Deb would enjoy the miniature containers of toothpaste, hand lotion, shampoo, and soap as much as I did.

Our parents agreed to extend our Kansas City visit an additional two weeks. Although Daddy and Janet had spent considerable time with me in the hospital, as a family we still had many activities to get in before Deb and I left.

Settled back at Daddy's house, I remained the center of attention entertaining friends and relatives with stories of my hospital adventures. Their curiosity and admiration helped keep my morale high, as I eased into my routine which would control the diabetes. I was proving to everyone just how responsible I could be.

By using the meal planning book I had received from the hospital dietician, I carefully measured my allotted servings of food. Daddy purchased a small scale and helped me weigh slices of meat for the evening meal. My diet allowed for 2,500 calories, which was not an overabundance for an active 11-year-old who was still many pounds underweight. I never felt deprived as I ate heartily from the four food groups. Janet bought me cartons of Diet-Rite®, the only sugarless soda pop on the market at that time, so that I would not feel left out. Whenever dessert was served, I never even thought of taking any. My father always took note of my abstinence and praised me for it. However, one night he surprised me.

After dinner one evening, I was helping to clear dishes from the table. On one trip to the kitchen I rounded the corner and saw Daddy standing there holding a big bite of chocolate cake in his hand. He was smiling as he moved the cake toward me and said quickly, "Here, Denny . . . don't tell anyone!"

I hesitated because I knew I was not supposed to eat sweets. But he was laughing and holding the cake up to my mouth, encouraging me to eat it before anyone saw us. The situation caught me off guard but, because I trusted Daddy, I went along with the game and ate the cake. Daddy was acting silly and it seemed so mischievous and fun. A couple of minutes later the exact situation occurred again, only this time it was with Janet. She was acting just as sneaky as my father had. I got the feeling they were in on this hanky panky together, so I complied and ate the bite she offered.

"Cheating" is a term used with diabetics to denote the eating of sweets or other foods not allowed on the diet, or eating larger portions of the permitted foods. To "cheat" had never occurred to me. There had been no forbidden fruit to tempt me at the hospital, and the staff stressed that I should stay away from sugary foods. The after dinner game of sneaking desserts went on for several nights and nothing bad happened to me. I felt as good as ever. What seemed like innocent fun was actually an unconscious signal to me that no price apparently has to be paid for occasionally eating an extra bite of food.

It was not that my father encouraged me to overeat. Just the opposite was true. He was the only one who supported me in awkward situations when I could have chosen to be like others and just eat anything I desired. He made me feel noble for refraining from sweets. In particular, I remember one hot evening when the family drove to a Dairy Queen®. I felt like a little martyr as I drank a carton of milk while the rest of them ate ice cream cones. I tried not to think of the ice cream they were enjoying as I said, "It's not what you eat that's important, it's what you are." Daddy acknowledged the words that I had uttered so profoundly. He added that diabetes is actually a blessing in disguise because I had to exercise and watch what I ate, whereas other people might not be as careful. I was strong and brave when he spoke like that and I felt special.

With others, however, it wasn't the same. Instead of pride, there was a sense of shame. An example of this occurred when we were all invited to a friend's home for dinner. The main course was to be spaghetti. I overheard the hostess asking Janet if I could eat spaghetti or did I need something else. Janet said I would not require special food, but that she would have to measure my serving. For some reason, I was very embarrassed by this and my eyes welled up with tears. In this situation I was the oddball being singled out from the other kids.

By contrast, I did not feel removed from my peers when it came to taking insulin shots. Instead, I took advantage of this difference between me and my friends in order to get personal recognition. Whereas for some children, getting a shot or watching someone else get a shot can be a frightening and even traumatizing experience, for me there was never any aversion to it. It was only a matter of making myself complete the procedure.

I learned to give myself shots while still at the hospital, as soon as the I.V.'s were removed from my arms. One morning a nurse told me there was something she wanted me to try out. In her hand were an orange and an insulin syringe. By using the orange to represent my skin, she demonstrated the proper technique for giving an injection. She held the syringe at an angle and quickly jabbed the needle into the fruit. She repeated this several times. When she let me try it, I thought it was great fun. She then left with instructions for me to practice, which I did for hours on both the orange and a rubber ball until I was comfortable with the action.

During another session, I learned how to fill a syringe with insulin. It is a simple, but exact procedure. The first step was for me to gently roll the insulin bottle between my palms. The rolling action mixes the contents without forming bubbles. Next, I pulled back the plunger to the number on the syringe barrel which indicated my correct dosage. Then

I inserted the needle into the bottle and pushed the plunger to move the air from the barrel into the bottle. This equalized the air pressure and prevented the formation of bubbles. Injecting a small amount of air into my body would not hurt me, but bubbles can prevent a correct dosage from being measured.

When the time came to solo with my first shot, Daddy and a nurse were there to cheer me on. The nurse pinched up an inch of skin on the upper outside of my left arm, so that the needle could penetrate the fat just underneath the surface. The shot could have been painful if the insulin were injected into a muscle. I felt a bit nervous and anxious to please. Not only was it important for Daddy to see how quickly I could learn something new, but that he also be proud of my brave, grown-up attitude. When I actually put the needle into my arm and pushed the insulin in, I was surprised at how easy it was. I completed all the steps without a flaw! I could not help smiling as my audience, who had been anxiously watching, praised and congratulated me. From then on one of the nurses always observed but did not help as I administered all my own insulin.

The transition from hospital setting to home environment for taking shots had been both an opportunity to show off and a test of courage. I had to give myself two shots a day, one before breakfast and one before dinner. The evening shot was no problem because, as at the hospital, I was never alone. I always asked Deb, Janet, or Daddy to pinch up the skin on my arm while I put the needle in. I doubt any of them realized how much their presence helped me. I wanted them to appreciate my courage and maybe even feel a little sorry for me.

Frequently several neighborhood kids gathered around me for the event and I could not disappoint them. The kids had mixed reactions. Some were fascinated and wanted to hold my arm for me or even give the shot to me, while others could not bare to watch and closed their eyes. Still others watched with nervous curiosity, ready to turn away if the sight proved too unbearable. Whatever the reaction, they were all so impressed.

Another matter entirely was the morning injection. At 7:30 A.M., when I was supposed to take the shot, my father had already left for work and my sisters and Janet were still asleep. Feeling very alone, I often thought of waking one of them up so I'd have that extra needed inspiration.

The site for these shots was the upper front portion of either of my thighs, where I could pinch the skin with my left hand while holding the syringe in my right hand. Many a morning I sat on the edge of our double bed, with Deb sleeping only inches away, needle poised over pinched skin. My right hand would shake nervously as I made feeble jabbing motions, for as long as half-an-hour, scared to insert the needle. Finally, out of exhaustion I completed the act. I never shared my fear with anyone.

As a result of this early hesitation, I developed a ramming technique that causes most onlookers to cringe. I never have been able to start with the needle close to the skin and gently puncture it. Instead, I more or less take a running leap, jabbing the needle from more than an inch away. Attempts to tone down my dramatic entry have failed. It seems to be the only way for me to get the job done.

The hospital nurses emphasized that I should rotate the injection site from arms, to stomach, to legs, to hips. This rotation prevents the appearance of small, unattractive pockets in the skin. It was some time before I was courageous enough to try either my hips or my stomach. When I did, I found the hip shots to be difficult because of the awkward angle required to insert the needle. Many shots in my hips were painful when the needle went into muscle.

During my first attempt at a shot in my abdomen, I scared myself by accidently sticking the needle into my thumb. The only resulting injury was the puncturing of a tiny blood vessel, but I quickly learned to be more careful. I found the stomach an easy, inconspicuous area for an injection.

With the exception of my father, I failed to persuade any members of my immediate family to give the shots to me. I would patiently explain the procedure, and assure everyone that they could not hurt me, but they could not bring themselves to try it. Poor Deb even felt uneasy about holding up my skin, and she often let go before I had pushed the insulin in. It was always a pleasant relief for me to have someone else do the jabbing, but it was actually in my best interest when no volunteers came forward. Years later, I was shocked to find college-aged diabetics who still had their mothers giving them insulin shots. I was glad for my independence in that area.

The needle of an insulin syringe is very short and sharp. A shot does not hurt at all if the skin is pinched up, when the needle is inserted at a 45 degree angle, and when the plunger is not pushed too rapidly down the barrel. Occasionally there will be pain if the rules are not followed. Nurses frequently use a poor technique and unnecessary pain occurs. As a general rule, however, insulin shots are nothing more than a minor inconvenience.

Another responsibility I had to assume that summer was urine testing. While in the hospital, urine testing was just another activity to keep me busy for a few minutes. I learned the procedure but never comprehended the reason for testing. I thought it was something I just had to do. I was ignorant in an innocent sort of way.

I was taught the old Clinitest® method in which a tablet is dissolved in a mixture of urine and water, and the color change is noted. I imagined myself a little chemist at work with my test tube, eye dropper, and tablets. It was intriguing for an 11-year-old to watch the solution in the tube bubble and change colors. This test, which I had not understood, is used to measure the amount of sugar in a sample of urine. This, in turn, is an indirect way of determining the amount of sugar in a person's bloodstream at a given time. When the amount of sugar in the blood gets too high at any one time, the excess spills into the urine to be eliminated. Therefore, the urine test served as a gauge of how the diabetes is being managed. I was to carry out this test four times a day: upon rising, before lunch and dinner, and again at bedtime. The results were recorded on a chart which I showed to my doctor on office visits.

The final part of my new role as a diabetic was learning about the occurrence of insulin reactions in my body. Reactions were an interesting but mysterious phenomena to me and my family. They were explained to me in a very superficial way by one of the nurses at the hospital. I was told briefly how I would feel physically — strange and shaky — and what to do — drink orange juice immediately — but, I was in no way prepared for any emotional or psychological impact. That I would find out on my own. When I asked the nurse how I would know when I was having a reaction she replied, "You'll know!"

This vague explanation left me wondering if a reaction would be as a mere tap on the shoulder, or if it would be like falling down a flight of stairs.

Luckily for me my first reaction happened while I was still in the hospital. I was alone at the time and began to feel unusually warm. I held out my hand and saw that it was trembling. I decided that this must be it and switched on my call light, telling the voice on the other end that I thought I might be having a reaction, but that I wasn't sure. Within minutes a nurse carrying a glass of orange juice rushed into my room. She handed it to me and watched to see that I drank it all. She stayed with me the few minutes it took for my symptoms to go away, and she kept asking me if I was all right.

All in all my first reaction was not a dramatic experience. Later, I got a kick out of showing others how my hand quivered when I was having one. I was a weird kid!

As with the other aspects of my diabetes, my understanding of insulin reactions was somewhere in the future. The technical name for what was happening to me was hypoglycemia, or "low blood sugar." This means the body is losing its delicate balance of glucose (sugar) in the bloodstream. Glucose serves as ready fuel for the body. What happens during hypoglycemia is the opposite of what took place when the first symptoms of my diabetes appeared. At that time, the amount of sugar in my blood was extremely high. During hypoglycemia the body is "reacting" to a too low amount of sugar in the blood.

This condition develops for a number of reasons. Too much insulin, too little food, too much exercise, or a combination of these factors are the most common cause for hypoglycemia in a diabetic. When the level of sugar drops too low, a diabetic's body cannot convert stored energy, such as fat, quickly enough to restore the balance of sugar to normal. This in turn results in the symptoms of an insulin reaction. These symptoms can be any of the following: unusual perspiring, fatigue, impatience, irritability, trembling, headache, hunger, gradual loss of fine motor skills, and, if not treated, eventual coma. All but the last symptom are warning signs an individual can notice and treat before he reaches the coma stage.

The body is amazing in that it begins to pour sugar into the bloodstream even after a person goes into a coma. However, this is done very slowly and it is a critical situation to be in. A person with a healthy pancreas (organ in the body which produces insulin, the hormone needed to turn food to energy) automatically maintains a perfect level of sugar at all times and under any conditions. This person can go for days without food and, although feeling weak, still be able to function. This might not be healthy, but it would not necessarily be dangerous, and probably not fatal. A diabetic has to work hard to keep the level of sugar in his body as close to normal as possible by controlling diet, insulin, or other medication, and exercise.

Early in my life as a diabetic, any reactions were mild and easily controlled by drinking fruit juice or by eating a few sugar cubes. I would feel uncomfortable telling someone I was having a reaction because I feared that they would think I was making an excuse to eat sweets. In those days my knowledge of reactions was so minute that I did not have any idea what brought them on. I gave the matter little thought because reactions occurred so rarely.

All the new events in my life were very abstract to me. I never thought that diabetes would change my life that much. My days were filled with play and my new duties, and I was aware only of the fact that our vacation with Daddy was flying by. What the future held was of no concern. I was young. It was summertime, and—like any child—I lived for the present. It was a brief moment of innocence.

Chapter Four

ENEMIES AND ALLIES

BACK IN Albuquerque, my family consisted of all females: me, Deb, Mother, Grandma, my four-year-old sister, Lisa, and our black Schnauzer puppy, Sophie. Grandma did the shopping and cooking and helped take care of us girls, while Mother worked as a typist.

My sisters and I were very close to Mother. She was active and vivacious and often did special things with us like taking us out for banana splits whenever friends spent the night at our house. It is a challenge for a young woman in her thirties to work full time and raise three daughters, but Mother met that challenge with much enthusiasm. Knowing we lacked a father in our daily lives, she made up for it in every possible way. She trusted us with responsibilities at a young age, and saw to it that we always had sharing times together, whether it was going out for hamburgers on Friday nights after Mother got her paycheck, or going to amusement parks, or just spending a Sunday evening at home watching one of our family's favorite T.V. programs, "Gunsmoke."

Mother never did anything half way. The year she took over as leader of the Campfire Girl troop which Deb and I were members of, everyone agreed it was the best year we'd had. She helped us earn our beads in unique ways and planned memorable field trips. She even surprised the troop one summer by transforming our garage into a Campfire meeting place, complete with brightly painted walls and animated pictures of pretty Indian maidens in full, ceremonial costume. We were all so proud of that garage!

Shortly after Deb and I returned home from our vacation, Mother showed me where she had cleared off one of the bathroom shelves just for me. It was to be used for all my paraphernalia: syringes, cotton balls, alcohol, and materials for testing urine. Giving me an entire shelf was quite an indulgence, considering five of us shared the small room. I hugged Mother for thinking of me. After I arranged all my supplies on the shelf, I taped a sheet of paper to the inside of the cabinet door on which to record test results.

The syringes I used were made of glass and had to be sterilized in boiling water after each use. I was meticulous about keeping the syringe clean. Only the barrel and plunger had to be boiled. Only the needle was disposable and discarded after one use. When plastic syringes which were completely disposable came onto the market, I could not believe how easy and non-time consuming taking shots became.

At seven cents each the syringes were not individually expensive, but after a long period of time the cost was considerable. By purchasing 500 at a time, my father could get them wholesale, and he kept me supplied with syringes for the first couple of years. He would mail me an entire 500 at one time. Initially, the arrival of the boxes caused momentary jealousy among my sisters, when the mailman announced, "Package for Denise Bradley!", but any envy was short-lived when the contents proved to be only "stuff for Denise's diabetes" and "nothing fun." To me, though, they were always an acknowledgment from Daddy that I and my diabetes were important.

After using one of the new syringes, I had to remember to replace the cap on the needle and then break it off from the barrel. This was to prevent its reuse by me or anyone else. Sometimes Deb and I used the harmless little barrels for miniature squirtguns. Lisa, in her own creative way, used the plastic parts encasing each syringe to make furniture and accessories for her Barbie dolls.

Lisa was calm about my taking shots, and she willingly held my arm and pinched up the skin for me. Grandma, like Deb, helped only reluctantly, while Mother couldn't bear to be in the same room whenever I gave myself insulin. More often I enlisted Deb's assistance, perhaps in an attempt to involve her in that part of my life.

Deb and I played out the remainder of the summer and then entered the sixth grade. It was the fall of 1963. My first school year with diabetes always stands out in my mind because of the assassination of President Kennedy. I remember the day so clearly. One of my girlfriends took the news very badly and ran around the playground screaming that the Russians were going to take over the United States. Despite her lack of authority for such information, we were all quite upset, some even to the point of tears. School was let out early that day, and I raced home on my bicycle to tell Grandma the news. Of course, she had already heard.

The year went smoothly for me. Mother informed my teacher that I was diabetic and briefed him on the symptoms of an insulin reaction, in the event I had one at school. I carried sugar cubes in my lunch box as a precaution, but rarely needed them.

Only a few close girlfriends were aware of my diabetes. I was reluctant to annouce the fact to just anybody. The ones who did know assumed that giving myself shots and refraining from eating sweets was all there was to taking care of my predicament. As a result, I had difficulty in explaining such concepts as urine testing or insulin reactions. Since even I did not comprehend the total picture of my disease and how to manage it, those around me got a particularly distorted version of what it was all about.

This misunderstanding was a source of friction one weekend when my friend Henrietta and I were attending a church picnic. We were having a great time and had worked up quite an appetite. Eating was the main event, and tables of food were everywhere, set up smorgasbord-style. I ate extra servings of salads and vegetables, while steering clear of potato chips, baked beans, and marshmallows. Henrietta suggested we go back for more hot dogs. I declined by telling her that I could not eat any more meat for that meal. Teasingly, she replied that of course I could eat more because hot dogs did not have any sugar in them. My feeble attempts to explain what little I knew about the chemistry of food only served to anger her. She insisted that hot dogs did not taste sweet and could not possibly have sugar in them. We argued back-and-forth, with neither convincing the other.

Watching Henrietta storm off to get her fourth hot dog, I had felt frustrated and confused. What she said made sense to me, while all I could do was repeat what adults had told me. Why didn't she just believe what I was telling her and not get mad.

After Henrietta had her fill, we rejoined the games and had soon forgot our differences. I concluded that the less said to friends about diabetes, the better.

The only time diabetes was openly talked about was at the doctor's, and those occasions had been infrequent as well as superficial. Mother had made arrangements for me to be under the care of a physician at a nearby clinic. We met with him every three months. He was a soft-spoken and reserved man who did make an effort to educate Mother and me. We would sit in his office and watch him draw diagrams on a small chalkboard, while listening to the terminology of diabetes. When he asked us if we understood, we both nodded our heads up-and-down, even though we were not comprehending a word. Unfortunately, we were too intimidated to confess our ignorance. Since he always said I looked healthy and gave me a good report, we assumed that I must be doing something right. As long as he knew the technicalities of diabetes, Mother and I thought everything was taken care of.

Aside from visits to the doctor, I gave my diabetes little thought. I was too busy being an active child, which — unbeknownst to me — was the reason I was in such good health. My intake of daily calories may have been large, but I ran them all off. Every day my sister and I walked or rode our bicycles to school. Often we stayed afterward to practice track and field events, or we would go home and roller skate, play tether ball, or play hide-and-seek with neighborhood friends.

When our year in sixth grade ended, our contented world was upset by news from Mother. She informed us that for the next three years we would be attending a private church school. She wanted us in a stricter educational and social environment than that provided by public schools. The new school was located downtown in an unfamiliar neighborhood. Deb and I felt abandoned because all the kids we knew would be going to either of the two public junior high schools in our area. We couldn't believe Mother would take us away from our friends. How could she be that mean? In retaliation, Deb and I argued, cried, threw fits, and even secretly called our father, from a pay phone, and pleaded with him to help change Mother's mind. Daddy was sympathetic and said he would talk to Mother and assured us that she was not doing it to punish or hurt us.

Our show of disappointment was to no avail. Mother was firm, but she did agree that we could return to public school if we tried the new place for one year and found we didn't like it. We were somewhat appeased and directed our thoughts to the following year, when we would rejoin our old friends in eighth grade. We hated the new school before we saw it and throughout the summer, kept hoping that someone or something would intervene to change our inevitable future.

No sooner had the school year begun, when our fears and resentment subsided. As is typical with children, we quickly adapted to the change and soon became involved in our new surroundings. Mother had been wise in sending us, and needless to say, we spent some of our happiest school days there.

One of the things Deb and I liked most about the new school was the fact that there was only one class per grade level. This meant that after being separated six years, we were again in the same classroom. Our togetherness gave us emotional support during those awkward first days and, as a team, we easily made new friends. We were really close to two of the girls and, as usual, there was no pairing off. We were a foursome.

Because of the limited number of students in each age group, competition between the sexes was less. I was surprised and pleased to have boys paying attention to me. I got sideways glances, whistles, notes, and phone calls, and even heard through gossip that certain boys liked me. That new taste of flattery was a boost to my ego and, more than anything, helped influence my attitude toward the new school.

Upon entering junior high, Deb and I left our childhood behind us in many respects. We now had the responsibility of riding the city bus to and from school. Also, what was formerly game time at recess, now became gossip and boy-watching time. Instead of running around after school, that playtime now became time for conversation. Since our new friends lived in different parts of the city, the telephone became invaluable as we spent hours analyzing and speculating about hairstyles, dress lengths, and love interests. We also devoted more time to doing homework and watching television than we had in the past.

This period of budding self-awareness and social maturing was exciting for both of us, and we moved into each new day with anticipation. Feeling healthy and energetic, I was happy to be at that point in my life.

Two incidents occurred during the seventh grade, which, although puzzling, took on no real significance for me or my family. The first incident took place when our class at school was taking achievement tests. As we finished each section of the answer booklet, we were to put our heads on our desks and wait for further instructions. After a particular section, I put my head down. The teacher walked over to me and quietly asked if I had finished all the questions. I said yes and put my head back down. After the following section, I was questioned again, and I began to wonder why the teacher had singled me out.

Later, when the tests were being scored, I was called into the principal's office. He showed me sections of the booklet where I had completed only a third of the questions. I had no recollection of having done this and said so to him. Fortunately, he knew I was diabetic. He phoned Mother to discuss the situation, and together they determined that the diabetes must have had something to do with it. I was allowed to retake the tests.

Months afterward, a group of us students were passing around school annuals for signatures. During recess, I heard through the grapevine that one of the ninth grade girls was angry with me. I was perplexed as to why and asked a friend what I could have done to annoy the girl.

My friend discovered that when I was given the girl's book to sign, I had instead scribbled all over the page. I was shocked, but again, had no memory of the incident, so I could not testify as to my guilt or innocence. I approached the older girl and asked to see her book. Sure enough, there were ink scribbles covering the page which held my picture. Feeling very embarrassed, I apologized to her and explained that I had not done it on purpose. She acknowledged my sincerity and forgave me.

Mother was curious when I recounted the story to her. We ruled out insulin reactions because I had not experienced any of the usual symptoms. When no further suspicious behavior followed, we soon put it out of our minds. I now suspect that in both cases I had actually experienced low blood sugar and suffered from partial, temporary blackouts as a result.

My changing lifestyle was beginning to affect me in many ways. Even though I attended gym classes daily at school, the amount of physical activity I participated in was gradually reduced. I began to feel hungry all the time, and I no longer found my food allotment satisfying. What I did not know at the time, was that exercise helps suppress appetite. As a result, my increasing inactivity was of no help to me.

The most difficult time for me was after school when my small snack only teased my stomach. My meal planning book contained a list of "free foods," which could be eaten in any amount at any time. The list included bouillon, pickles, and vegetables such as celery and lettuce. Not real appealing to a hungry teenager. If I complained to Grandma about my hunger, she would tell me to eat lettuce. I did that, sometimes consuming half a head of the stuff in hopes that quantity would make up for quality.

However, the leafy greens were not fulfilling, and I began to hang around the kitchen in anticipation of dinner. By this time of the day, Grandma had usually cooked up a pan of spaghetti or some other dish for the main course, and I would help myself to two or three spoonfuls, just to tide me over. It was easy to begin to lose track of the number of spoonfuls I ate.

Since I was in the kitchen so often, I asked Grandma if she would teach me to cook. My interest pleased her, and she readily took me on as her protégé. Soon I was learning her tricks of the trade and used her method of cook-as-you-go. This method which used recipes only as basic guidelines relies on the taste buds to do the rest. Of course, I approved of this method and frequently taste-tested whatever I prepared.

Deb, on the other hand, hated to cook and did not understand the pleasure I derived from it. This was our first real diversion of interests. Generally, we still had the same likes and dislikes in other areas. Grandma introduced us to sewing, which we both loved. We began to sew many of our own clothes. We always sewed the exact same patterns and used the same fabric and as usual, wore identical outfits on the same day.

Our custom of always dressing alike came to an abrupt end, after an amusing but embarrassing incident at school. Deb, the two girls we chummed with, and I decided to make identical dresses. We chose the same pattern number and agreed to buy material which matched the lavender and white-checked fabric of the dress illustrated on the pattern envelope. When we completed our sewing, we planned to wear the dresses on a designated day, thinking it would be fun to look like quadruplets.

The day finally came. Deb and I arrived first, looking just alike. When the other girls made their entrance, we all burst out laughing. The four of us did not match as we had planned. We discovered that the others had used different shades of the main color, ranging from light lavender to dark purple. Also, some of the dresses had ruffles and some did not, and the sleeves and hems were various lengths. All of a sudden our grand idea seemed ridiculous. Although we were greatly amused by the mistake, we had not expected to be laughed at and teased by the other kids. We could hardly wait for that school day to end.

Deb was more than embarrassed by the incident and suggested that we begin wearing certain dresses on different days of the week. I would have preferred to keep dressing alike, but I sensed that she was taking a stand on the issue and so I agreed. It felt funny dressing differently from her, and I found myself making continuous comparisons of how we each looked. It was a big change for us, an attempt to be different . . . but just a *little* different.

Meanwhile diabetes was not a major issue between us and seldom came up. It was just an extra factor that I had to deal with and which she did not. However, the following incident served to bring it to the forefront.

Deb, Lisa, Mother, and I were driving home from an early morning church service one Sunday. Mother pulled into a supermarket parking lot and told Deb and me to run inside and buy something for lunch, emphasizing that we could pick out whatever we wanted. We eagerly climbed out of the car, as we loved the responsibility of shopping on our own. Inside the store I pushed the cart, while Deb located the items we had decided upon. Suddenly, Deb hollered at me that I was about to run the cart into a display of canned goods. Startled by her outburst, I redirected the cart and continued slowly down the aisle. I thought I moved cautiously, but every few moments Deb would yell, "Denise, watch out!" I began to realize that I was weaving back-and-forth and that my vision was blurry.

The next thing I knew I was sitting on a table somewhere and an unfamiliar man was asking questions while repeating my name over and over. I was annoyed because I could not figure out what it was he wanted from me. Glancing down at myself, I noticed that I was wearing my good Sunday outfit, an off-white jacket and matching skirt, but I was unable to assimilate that knowledge with anything going on around me. As my mind began to clear, I was reassured to discover that Mother was sitting nearby. A glass was thrust into my face and I was told to drink its contents. A few minutes later I became conscious of what was going on.

The man questioning me identified himself as a doctor and explained that I was in a hospital emergency room. He asked me if I had taken the correct amount of insulin that morning. He wanted to know what my dosage was and what I had eaten for breakfast. I answered in slow, deliberate words. The doctor spoke to Mother for a few moments and then left. Mother asked how I was feeling. I said okay, but that I didn't understand what was happening. She put her arm around me, said that she was glad I was all right and that she would explain everything later.

After a 20 minute wait, we were informed we could leave. As Mother and I approached our car, I was bewildered by the fact that Deb and Lisa were not there waiting for us. I had assumed we came to the hospital directly from the grocery store. Once inside the car, Mother started to explain. Her story was incredible.

Apparently Deb and I made it safely from the store to the car. Deb's only comment to Mother was that I had acted kind of strange inside the store. When we arrived home, I stood in the living room, took clothes from a laundry basket and began throwing them all over the place. Everyone initially thought I was kidding around but when I continued my antics, they yelled at me to stop. I then ran outside to our garage, located at the back of the house, and proceeded to pound on the door while making loud, unintelligible noises. A terrified Deb ran after me, but she was baffled as to what to do. Mother thought to get some orange juice, and she came running out to the garage with it. She urged me to drink it, but I knocked it from her hand.

Mother then ordered me to get into the car so we could go to the doctor. Her words infuriated me, and I fought off any attempts to control me. My family had never seen me like this — acting like a wild animal — and they were frightened. Deb stood by me helplessly, while Mother raced into the house to phone a friend who lived in the next block. She asked her friend to send her husband over immediately to help get me to the hospital. He arrived in minutes and together they all managed to get me into the back seat of our car.

Mother's story dumbfounded me. I did not want to believe it, but she insisted that it all was true. I hated not being able to remember what had occurred over such a long interval of time. The doctor assured Mother that she had done the right thing in attempting to give me orange juice and getting me to the hospital. His diagnosis was that I probably had not eaten enough food to balance out the insulin I had taken that morning. He warned that I must never skip meals or snacks or forget to eat on time.

I detected a change in Deb after that eventful Sunday. Now she would question me anytime she saw me eating between meals. She would ask, "Are you supposed to have that?" She knew I was supposed to stay away from sugar, but she did not realize that eating snacks was necessary in controlling my diabetes. If I had already eaten my snack, I tried to assure her that my continued eating was the result of my feeling that a reaction was coming on. I started saying that whether or not it was true. She would then put her arm around my shoulder and say, "Okay, but please be careful, honey. I don't want something like that to happen again. It was *so scary.*"

Of course she had every right to feel apprehensive. After all, she didn't understand my diabetes any more than I did, and I think she feared the unknown above all.

With her watching me, I felt self-conscious and wasn't at all sure I liked this type of attention from her.

The pattern I had begun of eating an extra bite of food here and an extra bite there continued for several months. I went on believing that one more bite couldn't hurt and so, when I found myself overweight, I wondered where all the extra pounds had come from. How could I gain weight when I felt hungry all the time? Didn't being hungry mean that my body needed food? I was honestly confused.

Those added pounds signaled a change in my attitude toward myself. I was no more than 15 pounds overweight, which I did not consider to be a gross amount, but I felt fat. Psychologically, *feeling* fat can be just as devastating as *being* fat. Because I believed that fat people are associated with eating, I was now ashamed to eat in front of anyone, especially between meals. I was severely self-conscious about my weight. Instead of being motivated to change my behavior, I got in deeper. As my self-esteem plummeted, I became hungrier and ate more.

There were two students at school who were noticeably overweight. One boy, Paul, was chubby. At noontime, the other boys would take part of his lunch. Paul, trying to suppress his anger, would turn red with embarrassment. An overweight person in this situation seemed humorous to the other kids. Even I smiled, but inside I ached for him. I knew what he must be feeling, but I never voiced my empathy to anyone.

Patty, another student, was definitely fat. She was also fun and jolly like fat people are supposed to be. Patty took her weight matter-of-factly, eating a lot and not caring who knew it. If one of us, in a fit of anger, called her a pig, she would just call that person a name right back. At least she was open and honest about her love for food, and I never got the impression she was embarrassed by her size.

I remained close to Patty for several years, but I never confided to her about our mutual attraction for food. We were both too immature to recognize it as an emotional problem. I was thankful that my increased inability to control eating was not as physically apparent as that of Patty or Paul.

I became more brazen about the type of extra food I ate. I openly began to eat sweets, something I had never done before. More than ever, Deb observed my overeating and the weight I had gained. I think she sensed I was losing control of my situation, but she was at a loss as how to help me. She knew what I was doing was wrong but not why. Years later she would tell me that she never understood why I just didn't do what I was told when it came to my diabetes.

Her solution was to constantly reproach me. Her once mild reprimands were replaced with harsh accusations, as if she hoped the volume and tone of her voice would attract the attention of others and embarrass me into stopping. Instead of ignoring her, I became defensive and then, fueled her anger by eating more. We argued often, as her frustration with me and my frustration with myself spilled into other parts of our relationship.

My apparent lack of concern for myself confused Deb. I was deeply troubled by this partial break in our closeness, knowing it had been brought on by behavior I was unable to stop. Fearing that she could not, or would not, empathize, kept me from expressing my reasons to her.

Mealtimes at home became increasingly uncomfortable for me as the negative connotations of food grew. Even before a meal began, I was in turmoil. Grandma was strict about my diet and always prepared extra vegetables and diet desserts for me. For meals she would measure the exact amounts of these foods as dictated by my meal planning book. She then served them to me in separate sauce dishes, each with its own spoon. This meant that I would have from two to four bowls surrounding my plate at the dinner table. Since I was usually in the kitchen before dinnertime, I would take away the extra spoon when Grandma wasn't looking. Or, I would eat the contents of the bowls and remove them from the table before the rest of the family came in to eat. I was so embarrassed by those little bowls.

I suppose I believed that the bowls just emphasized the obvious difference between me and everyone else, that the others could eat what they wanted and I could not. I remained silent, though, because I knew how much care my Grandma put into preparing our meals and in teaching me to cook. I did not want her to think that I was ungrateful. Everything she did for me was inspired by love and concern for my health, so, why did I feel as I did?

During a meal if I took second helpings of anything but salads, Grandma quietly asked me if I was supposed to be eating the extra food. She never accused or yelled like my sister, but I was put in a Catch-22 position, for no matter what I answered, the question made me guilty. I felt humiliated as I turned red and mumbled some excuse. I did not resent her for asking, but myself, for taking the extra food. In any event, I still felt hungry and deprived.

I had to find ways to get more food. Often I volunteered to do the dishes so I could snack on any leftovers. It bugged me when Grandma would offer to help with the cleanup by putting the leftovers in the refrigerator—some help! I'm sure she saw me taking extra bites of food, but she said nothing. Paranoia must have set in, for despite her silence, I felt spied upon.

Mother remained my only true base of support during the emotional times with Deb and Grandma. She never yelled at or confronted me and rarely asked questions. I was so grateful for her silence. She continued to love and trust me despite my weight gain. Mother's trust made me at least want to try to change my lifestyle, while the others' reproaches only made me bitter.

I appreciated Mother's calm attitude toward my diabetes. Once she asked if I would like to attend a summer camp for diabetics, perhaps assuming that I could use help in accepting my limitations. Going to camp may have been the best thing in the world for me, but at the time, I scoffed at the idea and she did not push it. The thought of being lumped together with a group of diabetics offended me. I may as well have worn a sign declaring, "I'm different." Maybe I feared having to stick to a strict diet and the pressure scared me. I preferred to remain inconspicuous among my sister and friends, and to deal with any problems in my own way.

Mother's support for me may have stemmed from empathy as well as love, since she was having physical problems of her own. What I remember most about my junior high school years is how little any of us saw Mother. Late in the eighth grade, we began to see a different Mother than we had been used to. It began with her coming home from work extremely tired, eating a early supper, and going to bed for the rest of the night. I can recall looking out our living room window and watching her walk slowly up the sidewalk toward our house after work. She looked tired and weak, and I would get a sinking feeling in my stomach. Where was our cheerful, active Mother?

This routine continued for a year with none of us understanding her lack of energy. Deb and I resented Mother for being tired and in bed all the time. We missed her and had so much to share with her. I guess we took her lethargy personally. We could not comprehend anyone being constantly tired and only wanting to sleep.

We later learned that this period of Mother's life was the deceptively innocent start of a chronic disease more traumatic than mine, rheumatoid arthritis. When the diagnosis was made, we felt sorry for Mother and didn't want anything to be wrong with her. The symptoms gradually included stiffness in her joints and crippling in her hands.

Deb and I heard somewhere that some of the crippling effects of arthritis could be averted or postponed with exercise. We urged her to exercise or at least play the piano, which stood in our living room. Mother had always loved to play the piano, but now refused to play or exercise, because she said it hurt too much. Deb and I would get upset and tell Mother she wasn't even trying. We were being cruel without realizing it. I suppose we were fearful of what might happen to her.

About this time Grandma decided to return to her home in southern New Mexico. To help out Mother, Grandma took Lisa with her for the school year. After they left, Mother had a serious talk with Deb and me.

She said that with Grandma gone and with her in bed so much, we would have to take over the major duties of housecleaning and cooking, especially on weekends.

We were proud to accept the responsibility. It was something we could do for Mother. Grandma had trained us well to be thorough housecleaners and I looked forward to having a run of the kitchen, free of her watchful eyes. Little did I know that my new role as head cook would only add to my problems and help shape the "diabetic snowball" that was forming in my life.

Chapter Five

DUELLING DISEASES

TAKING OVER the kitchen was no trouble for me, and with Grandma gone I now had legitimate reasons to be in there more often. Upon getting home from school, I would change my clothes and head straight for what was becoming my favorite room. After eating a much deserved afternoon snack, I would start rummaging around for something to prepare for dinner. I loved it when our kitchen cabinets were well-stocked. Full shelves provided a type of security for me, as it was somehow easier to abstain from overeating if I knew there was plenty of food if I wanted it.

I steered away from baking since I knew I would not be able to control myself around an abundance of sweets. Also, I convinced myself that eating extra food was not so bad if the food was not cakes, cookies, or candy. Hamburger dishes and casseroles made from leftovers became my specialty. I preferred these dishes because I could do lots of sampling without any of it being missed, although it was a sure way to gain more weight — those goulash recipes slid down easily. If we were having pork chops, I could not eat one because then there would not be enough to go around at dinner. Since Mother insisted that Deb occasionally take a turn at cooking, I left this type of food for her to prepare. I received praise and recognition from the family for the meals I fixed. Of course, they did not know I usually made more of the food than what was served, having devoured the other portion in the process of cooking it. Their compliments made me feel good and pacified feelings of guilt I had about my sneaky eating habits.

Preparing and partaking of the evening meal was not the end of my indulging. Waiting till Mother had gone to bed, around nine or ten o'clock, and watching to make sure Deb was absorbed in homework or television, I would slip quietly back into the kitchen. If there were leftovers from

36

dinner, I would take a few bites of that. Sophie, who always trotted in after me, would watch my prowling with curiosity. As a token of appreciation for her silence, I gave her a few bites of food too.

I discovered bread was an easy food to sneak because no one noticed how many slices were in a loaf. Sometimes I would make as many as ten pieces of toast, piling each one with butter, cinnamon, and lots of sugar. I would down each slice before the next one was out of the toaster, having developed the habit of eating very fast to lessen the chance of being seen or reprimanded by a family member.

To wash down all the food, I chugged at least a quart of ice tea. Along with overeating, I was drinking more, about a gallon of liquid a day in a vain attempt to quench my unending thirst. What I did not know was that my thirst was *caused* by my overeating. In a diabetic's body, urine receives the overflow of sugar from the blood, thus increasing the volume of urine and making elimination necessary. Urination reduces the amount of body fluids, and there follows a sensation of thirst which is a signal to replace lost fluid.

At the time, I believed the exact opposite, that by drinking more, I could simply wash the sugar out of my body. With a twisted way of thinking I believed I was doing the right thing. I now know that this is a common misconception among many diabetics.

Even after these nighttime binges, my hunger was never satisfied, and I became obsessed with a desire to feel full, believing that if I could feel full just once, I would never have to overeat again. The only thing that would stop my eating was the unbearable bloating that occurred from my rapid intake of food and liquid. I thought I would burst. By this time I felt guilty and ashamed of myself.

Leaving the kitchen as quietly as I entered, I walked past Deb to the bedroom we shared. I shut the door behind me and lay on the bed. I had to lay on my back because it hurt too much to lay on my stomach. I would then sob uncontrollably and curse myself for not having any willpower. I would silently pray to God to forgive me and help me, fervently promising in return to never repeat what I had just done. After these periods of sackcloths and ashes I always felt better, renewed with determination and strength to overcome my obsession and stay on a diet. But it never failed, that the next day or a few days later, I would again repeat the same vicious cycle. I hated my body for feeling hungry, and I hated myself for having such little control. I believed my body—not my mind—was in charge of my life.

When Mother and I visited the doctor, he always emphasized that I eat exactly what was on my diet plan. I was too embarrassed to tell him how hungry I was, and I figured he would not allow any more food, so, rather than find out, I didn't ask.

This situation was ridiculous, of course, because I was already eating beyond my diet allowance, but I knew he wasn't aware of it. But I knew, and I was reminded of my eating binges every time I saw my reflection. I used to be skinny. What was happening to me now? To get my mind off my body, I would scrutinize my face for hours in the bathroom mirror to determine if I was pretty. I thought that if my face was pretty, I would somehow get by and not be rejected like some fat people were.

The now obvious physical differences between Deb and me were troubling. She was developing a nice shape while I gained unwanted weight. Everyone, including me, complimented Deb's figure, and I know this was important to her. In turn, she would tell me I had a good figure, but I knew that her words were said just to make me feel good. Others would tell me how nice I looked if they ever heard me talking about how much I wanted to lose weight or to be skinny. Although I trusted their flattery to be sincere, I believed it no more than I did my sister's words. The praises served only as a soothing concealment for what I did not want to face.

As for Deb, I think she was subconsciously glad she had a better shape, because it gave her some of the attention I had been receiving over the years for my diabetes. I began to feel jealous toward Deb, not only for her size, but also because she was apparently able to eat whatever she wanted, while still remaining thin, and she never seemed to be as hungry as I was. It amazed me that often she would not eat any food after supper and yet, she appeared satisfied.

With other curvaceous girls, it wasn't so much jealousy on my part as much as it was my idolizing them. I believed that each was more fortunate than me to be blessed with such a good figure. I rated myself a step lower than them because of my weight.

I did make a few attempts to rid myself of the undesired pounds. Back then, exercise was not the fad as it is today. There was no talk of cardiovascular exercises or aerobics. Exercise was associated primarily with serious athletes or heavy people trying to trim down, and it was not promoted as healthy activity for people in general. I thought exercise consisted only of calisthenics, which I participated in three days a week in gym class. None of us liked doing the exercises and having to wear the blue, bloomer-like gym outfits didn't help our attitude any.

To supplement my exercise program at school, I sent for a Jack

LaLanne record and exercise rope that were advertised on television, and I did brief workouts in the afternoons. Another time I got the booklet of Air Force Exercises and did them for awhile. But, in both instances, I gave up in despondency when no improvements were evident within a week or two. No one, including the doctors, ever told me that riding my bicycle, for instance, was exercise. All the literature on diabetes mentioned activities such as bowling, swimming, and tennis, but these were events I rarely had a chance to engage in. Anyway, I viewed sports as being fun, while exercise meant only monotonous hard work. It was never clear to me that sports were a form of exercise. The impression I got was that these activities were included in the pamphlets only to emphasize that diabetics could do normal things.

Even if I had exercised faithfully, however, I could not have taken off the extra weight, the reason being that I was ignorant of the fact that, simply, fat develops from eating more calories than the body burns. Still, I was constantly hungry and under the delusion that I was not eating *that* much. What I failed to understand was that regardless of the quantity I ate, it was more than my body required to function. Instead, I had convinced myself that my fat appeared for another reason — as a punishment for, not the result of, overeating. Exactly who or what was doing the punishing was not clarified in my mind, but, nonetheless, I believed it to be justly given.

On another occasion I secretly bought a box of Ayds® appetite suppressant and hid it in my dresser drawer. I really wanted them to work. I hoped the sweet, chewy cubes would magically take away my hunger, but of course it was not to be. They might have curbed my appetite had I given them a chance, but since I was expecting miracles nothing happened. A third of the way through the box I gave up on the directions and just ate them like candy, four or five at a time.

After I had been overweight for many months, my doctor suggested that I see a dietician for help with my diet plan. Mother accompanied me to the meeting with the dietician, who to my dismay, was skinny as a rail. It probably meant she knew her business, but I felt fatter than ever by comparison. She set up a new diet for me, but I seldom lost even a quarter-of-a-pound between visits and frequently gained instead. Feeling very embarrassed by this I would attempt to explain it away to Mother and the dietician. In a perplexed tone I would insist that I did not know where the weight came from because I really did not eat very much.

The dietician was passive about my weight gain. She never asked me

if I was getting enough to eat or if I was eating more than my diet allowed. She was full of information about what foods to avoid or cut
down on, but she lacked the intuition to see that I was not truly into the
program. She never got me excited or motivated about losing weight.

I knew that I could not diet, so I just played along by letting her think
I was trying. When she weighed me at the beginning of each visit, I
wished so much that I had lost several pounds, so I could surprise her
and Mother. But, a few hours after the appointment, I was overeating as
usual. I looked upon dieting as a slow, laborious process, while in my
mind I wanted to snap my fingers and be thin. Then dieting would be
simple because it seemed easier to stay thin, than having to lose weight.
I do not think the dietician had any idea of the torture I was going
through.

And what about my diabetes? Indeed, my obsession with eating was
affecting other areas of my life. For example, urine testing at which I
had once been faithful — was now something I despised. Instead of using
the former eyedropper method, I now used a convenient role of tape
which I could carry to school. I took fewer tests now because the color of
the tape always turned from yellow to dark green, which indicated a
high level of sugar in my urine. This occurred even when I had not eaten
for several hours. Angrily I would curse the results, knowing that the
Tes-Tape® did not lie. I rationalized about not taking the tests — the urine
sugar may be high, but at least I did not have to know about it. Each time
I saw my doctor he wanted to review my test charts. That was a problem
for me because I didn't keep any. So, guilty and desperate, I hurriedly
filled in a month or two of results before going to the office. I wrote down
anything that came to mind. Heaven knows what he made of it.

Also, many times before going to see my doctor, I'd go into the
bathroom and run vigorously in place for five or ten minutes. I hoped
this would reduce the sugar in my urine in case I had to leave a sample
at the doctor's. Of course, my efforts were in vain because physical exer-
tion burns up sugar in the blood, not in the urine.

I regretted not only skipping the tests, but the poor test results even
more. Behind all of this was my fear of the doctor or anyone else discovering my eating habits and forcing me to give them up. Unfortunately,
he never questioned me. All he wanted to know was the times I took
urine tests and if I had any insulin reactions. That seemed the most important to him, whether or not I was having reactions. I knew there was
little chance of that for I was eating constantly. I suppose I fooled him
because, except for the few extra pounds, I looked healthy, felt good,

and never had a cold or the flu. I often told people that if it weren't for the diabetes, I would be perfectly healthy.

As for Mother, she continued to work although her hands continually ached, and she tired easily. Lisa returned to live with us, but Grandma remained in Truth or Consequences. Too often, Deb, Lisa, and I were just rotten kids. We fought and argued after school and frequently called Mother at work to have her settle our disputes. Or, we would wait until she came home and then tattle on each other. This was the last thing she needed. Among the three of us, I was able to control my temper the longest. I could be angry when I wanted, but I tended to be more forgiving. Perhaps by projecting a sweet personality I could mask the secret behavior I shared with no one.

Lisa and Deb got into bitter arguments which often ended in knockdown, drag-out fights. It was a strain on all of us. One evening I went into Mother's bedroom to kiss her goodnight. She unexpectedly broke into tears and told me how thankful she was for me because I was such a good daughter and rarely caused her trouble. I was pleased to make her happy, but felt remorseful that each week I was eating away half of her hard-earned paycheck with my eating binges. For a moment I wanted to confess my transgressions to her, but the thought of disappointing her seemed worse than keeping them hidden. I kept silent.

This inability to control my eating, coupled with my need to conceal that inability, was woven into evey area of my life. I realize now that I was no different than a teenage alcoholic or anyone else addicted to drugs. My drug was food. The contemporary term for this disorder is "foodaholic" or "compulsive eater." But at the time I had no way of knowing that my food compulsion was a disease in itself, arising from an emotional or psychological problem. I thought of it only in connection with the diabetes and believed that if I was not diabetic, I would have had no difficulty in controlling my eating.

Even if I had shared my worries, I don't know if my family or the medical world could have dealt with them effectively, if at all. But, I can appreciate how counseling may have been helpful not only for me but the entire family.

Despite all this I somehow managed to do well in school. I earned the honor of being co-salutatarian at my ninth grade graduation, and I delivered a short speech to a packed church of friends and family. I was proud of myself for having done so well. It was an exciting way to leave junior high school.

There was one thing that made me apprehensive about going to high school—the breaks between classes. During junior high, my constant need for drinking fountains and restrooms had been easily met because the school was so small. However, the public high school Deb and I would attend had 3,000 students, and I worried that I would not have enough time to go to my locker and the restroom without being late for classes. It had been habitual for me to go to the restroom after every class, and if unable to do so for some reason, I was very uncomfortable. What a thing to be thinking of as I entered a new phase of my life.

Shortly after entering the new school, I settled into a rushed, but accommodating, routine for taking care of this concern. I quickly learned the location of every drinking fountain and girls' restroom, the shortcuts and least crowded hallways.

My physical calamities aside, there was an important event happening to Deb and me—learning to drive and getting our driver's license. For the two of us, being able to drive meant what it did to most teenage girls: being able to go shopping, running errands for ourselves and the family, feeling grown up, and going guy-watching, or, as we told Mother, "going to get a Coke®." We always did get something to drink, but we definitely had ulterior motives for going.

For me, though, learning to drive had a more subtle and dangerous meaning. Acquiring wheels was freedom from the watchful eyes of others and made it easier to hide my lack of self-control. I did all the things comedians joke about. I would drive to fast food places and order enough food for three adults, ordering it to go so it appeared I was buying the food for a group of people. I also bought several drinks to enhance the cover-up. Or, I would order food at one place, drive to another a mile down the street and innocently reorder the same items. How polite I was to the counter girls and guys who were my unwitting partners in crime.

Many times I purchased a dozen doughnuts and then drove around aimlessly while I ate every one of them. I even stopped at garbage bins located behind stores to discard the empty boxes, thus destroying any evidence. I was shocked at my own behavior and thought I was the only one in the world who did such things.

My best girlfriend and I would go to a restaurant on Saturday afternoons to have a snack and to talk. I drove to her house to pick her up. Dorcas, my petite, slim friend usually ordered ice cream, but I always ordered "good food"—a ham and cheese salad and ice tea. Afterward, I dropped her off at home and then drove directly to a drugstore to buy a few candy bars, which I gobbled up before reaching home.

When I was out with Deb and friends to football or basketball games, I kept up my front. After the games we'd cruise Vip's Big Boy, which was our school's most popular weekend hang out. When we stopped for food, I never ordered Cokes or other sugared drinks, always ice tea. It was easier for me to have the others pity or admire me for sticking to tea than it was to have them question me or give me the evil eye. I knew these rebellious acts were no better just because they were hidden, and I suffered terribly knowing how hypocritical I was. But, for some reason, even that guilt was never enough to stop me. The compulsion was as strong as ever and being mobile just made everything that much easier to get away with.

Our need and desire for spending money kept Deb and me busy during high school. We did babysitting, housecleaning, and took in ironing to earn all our own money for the next four years. We got most of our jobs by word of mouth from satisfied customers because we were both reliable workers. Driving allowed us to take more jobs and make more money.

As in other areas of my life, my food addiction followed me into the job market. It seems that all my jobs were either directly related to food or put me in a position where I could easily get it. While babysitting I was never timid about eating other people's food. Sometimes the parents would leave food out for me, food such as potato chips and pop. I ate modest amounts of these foods. After the kids were in bed, the second half of my Dr. Jekyll and Mr. Hyde personality took over, and I would spend an hour or more in the kitchen going through the refrigerator and cabinets to check the available stock. I snacked on anything and everything, from cereal to leftovers to jellies and ice cream toppings. I took only a few bites of each food just as I had been doing at home for years.

I was always neat and clean and left no evidence of my raid on a kitchen. Without exception I picked up the house and washed dirty dishes. I got to the point where I remembered other people's kitchens and the type of food they kept on hand. If there was not much food at a certain house I would not want to work there again. Was I ever surprised and disappointed my first evening at one home. When I checked out the refrigerator, I found it filled with nothing but juice and fresh carrots. I found out later the family was vegetarian!

For several summers I had permanent babysitting jobs lasting from one to three months. The jobs involved taking care of children, cleaning, and some cooking. I preferred to have the kids playing outside so I could be alone in the kitchen. If one of them walked in and saw me eating,

I blushed with embarrassment. I would make a mental note to be more careful the next time. One nine-year-old girl I was in charge of followed me around like a puppy, and I wondered when I would be able to eat in private. Discovering that she enjoyed eating as much as I did was a relief. One day we both got carried away and polished off a half-gallon of ice cream. I'd broken one of my taboos about not revealing my greed for food, but since she had shared in the indulging, it didn't seem so bad.

With my housecleaning jobs customers were usually away at work when I did the cleaning. This suited me fine. I was thorough and fast, which meant I could spend more time in going through my favorite place. I had rules concerning my eating, such as: never finish off a dish, box, jar, or pan of any food, always leave a little and never open anything new. But, it was a whole other story if a package or container were already open. Both of these strategies, I hoped, would disguise the fact that I was a glutton.

Why I had no qualms about eating the food of strangers or people I hardly knew, I do not know. If I had ever thought about it, I might have been disgusted. After all, anything could have happened. But, as an addict, I took it where I could get it.

During our senior year, Deb and I had our first opportunity to work at a real job, when a friend of the family helped us get hired at a chain of hamburger stands. We worked part time for the next three years. Talk about tempting fruit and the appropriateness of a name, Lota' Burger — I did a *lota'* eating there. It was my first time working directly with food, and I derived much security in this environment.

As soon as I became comfortable with my duties and the staff, I made no attempt to conceal what I ate. The fact that most of the workers were teenagers made it easier for me to be inconspicuous, because they ate all the time too. Even those who knew I was diabetic did not make a big deal about it. Lota' Burger employees could consume all the French fries, ice cream, and drinks they wanted, and each person was allowed one hot dog or hamburger per shift. I brought bottles of Tab® for snacks, but inevitably used it to wash down the free food.

Deb and I usually worked at separate stands, but one summer the only openings were at the same location. I was promoted to assistant manager by my boss, Jerry, who was also a good friend. Jerry was a hard worker who did not let our acquaintance get in the way of properly training me. She also had a hilarious sense of humor which kept all of us laughing and made her strict discipline more bearable.

It was sometimes an awkward situation when I was in charge, since

Deb spent half her time reprimanding me for eating. Also, I was dating one of the fry cooks, Richard. I will remember him because he provided a positive diversion from food. He never scolded or nagged me about my snacking. Instead, he would grab me into the back room and kiss me. A subtle way to say, "Stop!" and a lot more effective than words.

I do not know whether eating filled a void in my life or was my way of rebelling against diabetes. What was certain was that I was powerless around food.

Chapter Six

FLASHING LIGHTS

MY DESPERATE lifestyle had become routine. To me, it was normal. Much of the time I was able to push my awareness of it to the back of my mind, as I involved myself in the everyday trauma of being a high school teenager. I loved shopping and going to movies, I cheered enthusiastically at school sporting events, enjoyed church activities, and waited hours in line to hear favorite rock-and-roll singers. I dated off-and-on and spent considerable time thinking about boys and making myself hopefully more attractive to them through constant attention to clothes, hair, and make-up. I was just beginning to explore the level of expressing my own opinions, as long as they were not too radical from those of my peers. I thought it was delightful to be a teen and among those who were on the verge of becoming adults. The happy times kept me secure in the knowledge that my life could only get better, and that my problems would eventually, somehow, come to an end.

I think I was more mature than other kids my age because of what I understood to be "coping" with my disease. In my mind, to cope was to accept, and it would be years before I realized the danger of my having projected such an accepting attitude. My attitude was fostered by many factors encompassing my diabetes. Although these influences were subtle, it was their constant repetition that gradually worked them into my budding self concept.

One factor was that I continued to be caught up in my cycle of non-control. As my behavior became habit, it seemed less of a crisis and more of just the way things were. The compulsion and guilt were still there but easier to tolerate. I was oblivious to the notion that I could live any other way.

Another factor was the negative atmosphere created by those around me, who thought they were speaking in my best interest. There was and is a stigma surrounding diabetes that is padded with worn-out, incorrect cliches. I first heard these cliches matter-of-factly from doctors whose words were repeated in the brief pamphlets on diabetes they gave me. They were retold to me constantly by nurses, lab technicians, medical receptionists, and acquaintances who had picked them up somewhere. Included in this barrage of so called wisdom were statements such as: diabetics take a long time to heal; diabetics don't heal normally; diabetics have eye problems; diabetics end up getting their legs and feet amputated; and, diabetics always get infections.

The trouble with these statements is that they are incomplete and therefore misleading. But, neither I nor others realized that. I got the impression that diabetes was a heavy cross to bear and that I had a lifetime of problems to look forward to. I often heard in sympathetic tones how unfortunate it was that I had diabetes at such a young age.

My doctor's warnings seemed trite and meaningless. He would tell me to avoid cuts and burns because I would not heal easily. That sounded ridiculous to me, as if I would intentionally cut or burn myself. They were just accidents that could happen to anyone, and it annoyed me that being a diabetic meant that I had to be more careful than others had to be.

When Deb and I began to shave, my doctor told me to use an electric shaver rather than a straight razor so that I would not cut myself. This irritated me because Deb and our friends used straight razors and I did not see the big deal in possibly getting a few cuts. But Mother bought a nice electric shaver for me and I agreed to try it. It did not leave my legs as smooth as a razor did and I switched back. I felt a little guilty using the razor and would rush through with my shaving. When I wasn't careful, I did cut myself.

Then, when I took up cooking and ironing, my tendency to rush led to frequent cuts and burns. It seemed to me that my cuts and burns healed quickly. I saw no basis for other's arguments, but they appeared anxious to pin the label "slow healer" on me. The more the idea was drilled into me, the more cuts and burns I seemed to get. The power of suggestion was playing its part.

Because my family believed the cliches it was hearing, I received attention for every tiny wound. Their concern was a logical result of their belief in everything the doctor said. The family pleaded with me to be careful. At first I brushed off their concern and promised to be more cautious, but when their words began to sound like reprimands, I became defensive.

I cut my finger once too often while preparing dinner and Mother noticed. We got into a loud argument. I knew Mother was concerned about my health, but I was tired of being singled out. I insisted that I did not cut myself anymore than others did, but that didn't impress her. She said she forbid me to cook with a sharp knife. I yelled back that it was impossible to cook without one. Her response was, "Then you'll have to stop cooking altogether!"

This was getting into a sensitive area so I quickly dropped the subject. The taking away of cooking privileges would have been a disaster since I had to be around food. Gradually, I started using sharp knives when Mother wasn't around and I made it a point to be extra careful not to cut myself.

There was another area of home life where I had to learn to be careful. Deb and I dried our hair with bonnet type dryers that had plastic hoses attached. I dried my hair late at night while doing homework. The heat made me drowsy and I would fall asleep. An hour or so later I would wake up and discover I had little burns on my neck and arms. At first I showed the burns to Mother who implored me to be careful. But, as with the knives, when I had burnt myself several times, she forbade me to dry my hair late at night. I was angry but knew from experience not to say anything. For awhile I obeyed her order but soon I was using the dryer whenever I wanted. I concealed any burns from her. How I looked in school the next morning meant more to me than the fear of disobeying Mother.

Burns on my neck or the insides of my arms were easier to hide than burns on the outsides of my arms or cuts on my fingers. It got to the point where I hated to use Band-Aids® for fear they would draw attention to my cuts or burns. To me they were battle scars in my fight to be like others and I bore them bravely.

On one checkup at my doctor's, he suggested that I should not wear tennis shoes because they would not allow my feet to breathe. He handed me a pamphlet that warned about amputation. To a young girl who wanted to wear the fashion of the day, his logic escaped me. Just because I wore tennis shoes I may have to have my feet cut off? My feet looked and felt great and therein rested my belief. I did not stop wearing tennis shoes. If his logic evolved from the usual scare stories about diabetes, I was tired of hearing it.

During my junior and senior years in high school I began to encounter other health problems that were not as easily dealt with as minor cuts or burns. Because of what we had been hearing for years, my family and

I accepted these problems as inevitable consequences of my disease. I became the one in the family associated with sickness and physical calamities, and the one who would never be as healthy as other people. Secretly, I believed that this image was another punishment for my lack of control over food. With each new dilemma came the echos of my grandma's words, "Poor Denise, poor Denise."

Going through puberty I had the usual bouts with acne. Acne was a nuisance and embarrassing, but the onset of boils was humiliating, not to mention painful. I would get one or two boils at a time on various parts of my body — my ear lobes or inner thighs. The doctor told me that boils were infections inside the body that were seeking an outlet, and that they were common in diabetics. I quietly accepted this, but at the same time I was ashamed and felt like Dorian Gray whose secret sins were revealed to the world.

I also had a vaginal discharge and itching which caused me severe discomfort for months. Mother and some of my girlfriends confided that they also had this problem occasionally. If I had to have something else wrong with me, I was glad that for once it was apparently normal. My itching was so bad that between classes at school I would race to the nearest bathroom, go inside a stall and violently scratch my genital area for five minutes until I was burning with pain. The momentary pain helped me forget the itching, but momentary was all it was. All I could think about during classes was how many minutes until the next break.

If this itching was normal, everyone else seemed to be taking it rather casually. Washing up several times a day did not help. I finally told my doctor about it and he suggested I see a gynecologist. I was nervous about going because I did not know what to expect, but my discomfort was so great, that I quickly became immodest. The gynecologist informed me that I had a yeast infection, a situation not unusual with diabetic females. He prescribed medication and said the problem would clear up within a few days. I was depressed by the news of this being common in diabetic women, but also relieved when the itching went away. I did not know that common meant that the infection could reappear as quickly as it had gone away. When it did reoccur I was too embarrassed to ask the doctor for more medicine because I feared that he or my family might reprimand me for not taking care of myself.

Years later I learned from a book that one of the reasons diabetic women get yeast infections is because sugar is often present in their urine. Sugar is a breeding ground for the yeast fungi. The large amount of sugar always present in my urine was undoubtedly a contributing factor to my problem. Had I known this simple fact about urine sugar, I may have been encouraged to watch my eating in order to avoid the itching. But I was never told and never thought to ask. I believed that I had to endure the suffering, so I did.

The boils and other infections made me feel unclean, perhaps because, symbolically, they were the outward representation of what I had put into my body. In addition, there was another problem which I thought to be related to my diabetes, but which I later realized must have only been aggravated by the diabetes and not caused by it. The problem was bedwetting, a nightmare Deb and I shared. When it persisted into our teens, I took some comfort in the fact that we both had the condition and therefore diabetes could not be cited as the culprit. Since there were other instances of prolonged bedwetting in our family, we assumed it was hereditary and looked forward to the time we would outgrow it.

There was nothing more sickening than to wake up in the morning to the feeling of wet, sticky pajamas clinging to my skin. I always hoped I was dreaming or that I had perspired heavily during the night, but that was never the case. Deb and I were fortunate—and grateful—that Mother never scolded or belittled us about our problem, nor complained about having to wash so many sheets.

Our condition was a frequent cause of embarrassment. During junior high I dreaded spending the night with girlfriends. I would try very hard to stay awake so that I could keep going to the bathroom. One night I wet in Patty's sleeping bag but was too ashamed to admit it to her, so I said nothing.

After a time, my accidents were occurring much more frequently than Deb's were and none of us knew why. Mother's patience was taxed after I wet on our couch several times, because I fell asleep under the hair dryer. Mother said she was sorry but that she would have to forbid me to drink liquids after 6 P.M., to hopefully curb my wetting. Not drinking in the evening was agony for me because I continued to be perpetually thirsty. After refraining as long as I could, I would go to the bathroom and rinse my mouth with water, trying to quench my thirst and sneak a few drops in the process. After several days of this I started drinking as usual; Mother did not stop me.

Years later Mother had the couch recovered, but that did not cover up my painful memories. Deb grew out of bedwetting by the time we were seniors, although I continued until I was 20, still unaware that the constant presence of sugar in my urine added to the problem.

As to the forebodings about diabetics going blind, I paid little attention to them because my vision was excellent. My endocrinologist examined my eyes as a part of each checkup and occasionally I visited a doctor who specialized in eyes. I always got good reports. It was when I was in the twelfth grade that I was informed I may have the beginnings of an eye disease which occurs often among diabetics. Four specialists peered into my eyes with strange looking instruments and were intrigued by whatever they saw. The disease they suspected had a long impressive sounding name — diabetic retinopathy.

I was not the least bit disturbed by the diagnosis as my vision appeared to be flawless and I felt no pain or discomfort. True, I had recently purchased a pair of glasses for night driving, but that was normal enough.

The doctors in Albuquerque did not have the necessary sophisticated equipment needed to pinpoint the exact condition of my eyes. They suggested I see a doctor in Colorado Springs. If I decided to go, I had to prepare for several days of testing and even possible surgery.

While driving home I mused over what I had been told, and, to me, it seemed so dramatic — I might go blind. I thought of television shows about blind people and how brave they were, and how interesting their handicap with Braille, canes, and seeing eye dogs. These ponderings came and went as I wondered how to tell my family. How easy it is to be a martyr when one is preparing to go to war while still being safe and sound at home. That's how I felt when I announced the news to my family.

After a mild reaction on their part, none of us took it too seriously. Even more significant was the fact that none of us even questioned why I would be getting eye trouble now when I had never had it before. Instead we took it for granted that it was another inevitable side effect of diabetes. In the meantime, there I stood in front of my family with 20/20 vision.

Mother insisted we make the trip, anyway, to be on the safe side, and I agreed. Her friend Hank would be driving us to Colorado. I got a three day leave from school, which added to the importance of it all, as did the phrase "possibly have surgery."

Boy, were we surprised a few days later when the Colorado ophthalmologist told me that my eyes were fine and I could go home immediately. He confirmed the presence of the eye disease, which had not progressed to the point of needing treatment, inferring that action would have to be taken somewhere down the line. We decided to stay and sightsee for a few days. I was glad that nothing was seriously wrong with my eyes, but it just all seemed so anticlimatic.

Over the years, my family and I had come to expect physical changes in my body, believing the natural progression of any disease was toward the negative. By accepting what was "my due," my problems would soon be complicated to the point of no return.

Looking back, the most inexcusable part of this situation was the attitude of the doctors. By alternately being complacent about my condition and being fascinated by the changes in my body, they failed to look at the entire picture of my health. While they could expect, accept, and attempt to treat symptoms, they did not look for the root of the problems and literally could not see the forest for the trees. Now I know that there are no side effects to diabetes. There are only symptoms of uncontrolled diabetes. So, there I was with lights flashing in every part of my body warning me and my doctors that something was amiss.

I knew that I was fooling myself about being in charge of my diabetes, if only because of my overeating. The doctors, although not knowing of my private life, had the symptoms staring them in the face and yet they believed me when I said I was in control and doing all I was supposed to do.

I am amazed that not one of the doctors said to me, "Denise, here are the signs of good control and you do not have these signs. You have all these other problems and it just doesn't fit. Something has got to be wrong here." Despite the fact that I lied about my urine test results and about my eating, the effects of these actions spoke for themselves and should have been interpreted correctly. I guess the doctors thought they were doing their job by giving me pamphlets about diabetes or prescribing drugs to treat infections. But the spotting of trouble in psychological as well as physical areas could have made a big difference. I was too caught up in my disease to see what was going on, and I was in a sense crying out for help in the only way I knew how, but my calls went unanswered.

Chapter Seven

FREE TO CHOOSE

THERE WAS never any question that Deb and I would go to college. We had always loved school, made good grades, and planned that college would immediately follow high school graduation. Our choice was a small, private church school in the midwest, Midland Lutheran College in Fremont, Nebraska, which we chose mainly because two kids from our church were already enrolled there. We applied for admission and were not only accepted but also received financial aid in the form of grants and loans.

The months preceding our departure were filled with nervous anticipation for Deb and me. We were a bit apprehensive about the academic pressures of higher learning but had only great expectations for exciting social activities. We spent hours going through our clothes and personal belongings trying to imagine what we might need in future situations as college coeds. It was our first time making plans for a home away from home, so each decision was a major one.

Also, we made advance arrangements to be assigned to the same room in the college dormitory. After all, we had been rooming together all our lives and keeping it that way would be a type of security blanket for us in the midst of a new environment far from home.

August of 1970 arrived quickly and we could barely contain our excitement during the day-and-a-half car trip to Fremont with Mother and Hank. The older, stately-looking buildings of the campus surrounded by well kept lawns and flower gardens made a friendly first impression on all of us. After a few mix-ups we located the dorm Deb and I were assigned to. It was a small, more modern looking building adjoining the school cafeteria, where we would be working part time. It was comforting to have Mother with us as we got our first glimpse of the place where we would be spending the next four years of our lives. We were sad to see her and Hank leave the following day.

Our room was located on the second floor of Augustine Hall. I was thankful to see that it was only a few steps from a drinking fountain and restroom, but I had an uneasy feeling knowing I had to adjust to not having a refrigerator close at hand.

Being twins provided Deb and me with some identification and helped ease us into our new surroundings. Everyone remembers twins, even if they do get their names mixed up. Oddly enough, the twin label did not stick for long and soon others referred to us only as being sisters and not twins. Perhaps they thought it would be childish to refer to us that way, but I did miss the familiar ring of "the twins."

As for my having diabetes, I kept silent about it. The less others knew about me, in that respect, the more I liked it. There was no use taking a chance on having one of the girls treat me as my sister did, always reprimanding, always questioning. One person I did tell, the housemother, who was nice about it and let me keep my insulin in her apartment refrigerator.

My sister and I fell right into dorm life, loving every minute of it. I kept a schedule different from the one I kept at home, but I never gave it a second thought since I was having so much fun. At 10:30 each week-night and at midnight on weekends, the outside doors to our dorm were locked and all girls had to be inside. For most of us, unless there was an exam coming up, this was when our nightlife began. Some girl would make a huge batch of popcorn and we would gather in her room or the T.V. lounge to eat, gossip, and joke around. There were always birthday cakes or homemade goodies to snack on, and — if Deb wasn't looking — I snacked too. These were fun, relaxed times which drew us close like one big family.

Being Deb's roommate brought stress early on and it bothered me. Whatever our expectations about rooming together had been, little by little they disintegrated and we realized it had been a mistake. Deb was different toward me, not as friendly, and this was just a few weeks after we had been so close planning for our new experience. I suppose she was not acting differently than she had at home, but it was different than I had expected. I accepted that we were becoming individuals, but I did not understand what was wrong with retaining some of our closeness as sisters. We were more or less independent now, and I was surprised and hurt to find her continuing with her bossy role with me, not only about my eating, but on several other issues as well. For one, the way I kept my half of the small dorm room. My bed was often unmade and my desk forever strewn with papers. After all those years of straightening up other people's houses, I was lax about tidiness, but I couldn't see making such a big fuss. She repeatedly told me how messy and sloppy I was and I had the feeling she was actually more angry with me than the mess.

It did not help at all that I still wet the bed occasionally and she did not. I knew she empathized with me, but I felt childish now that she had outgrown it. I remember her waking up early and, if I had wet, she would race my sheets down to the basement laundry room and wash and dry them while getting ready for her first class. She was so afraid that one of the girls would find out about it. I hated still having the problem, but hated even more the reaction it caused in her.

It has been only in recent years that it has become clear to me what was happening to our relationship at that time. Deb had gone through more embarrassing and/or frightening episodes with my diabetes than she had ever cared to and probably wanted to set the record straight right away. At college, where we were surrounded by peers, she feared even potentially embarrassing situations. Unfortunately, she never told me about how she felt, perhaps believing that actions speak louder than words. I think she thought that because we were twin sisters, everything I was or did reflected on her, thus making her partly responsible. Maybe if I had been a younger sister my actions could have been chalked up to immaturity, but as twins the identification was more parallel. If I kept a messy room, she too must be a messy person. If I had weaknesses, she too must have them. After 18 years of being associated with me, she needed a break and for any bond between us to be less visible. What must have been hard on her was the fact that she did love me and did care what happened, and, therefore, could not be totally removed from me. But, at the time I was really puzzled. Her behavior never embarrassed me because I did not identify with it.

By being aware of Deb's attitude I was only mildly surprised to find her developing into a strong character in the dorm. I noticed with a sort of awe the way girls were drawn to her. They knew she was set in her ways and were amused by it. She was loud and funny and ready to have a good time. She liked being in a group and a group was naturally attracted to her. I also believe that having others around her served another purpose — it isolated her from me. I, in contrast, did not need a protective group around me. I was not as loud as Deb and, although not a loner, did not feel vulnerable if I was by myself.

We were in none of the same classes and we inevitably made separate friends outside the dorm. I could tell Deb was more happy being intimate with kids with whom I was merely an acquaintance.

Because it seemed the thing to do, I tried the drinking and partying scene for about the first month of school, but quickly tired of it. I found most of these gatherings gave me a sense of forced gaiety and a feeling that the other students were acting unnaturally. It was just as well that the drinking environment did not appeal to me — that was all my diabetes needed. I was content being a "foodaholic" even if I didn't know that I was. In fact, the only thing I ever looked forward to at any of these parties was the free food.

This type of socializing had not been a part of either mine or Deb's life during high school. Not that the opportunity wasn't all around, it just did not appeal to us and we were happy without it. Hence, I could not understand why she now thoroughly enjoyed these activities. I guess it was part of her search for self-expression and part of becoming a non-twin.

Deb was more popular than I in that she knew more of the students on campus and went to more social events than I. Because I was still 15 to 20 pounds overweight, I was a little self-conscious when it came to group functions. And, whereas Deb dated several guys, I went out with only a couple of guys before settling into a steady relationship with an upperclassman, whom I dated the remainder of my freshman year. Deb and I were becoming so opposite in temperment and activity that girls would say to us, "You're so different — I can't believe you're twins!" That certainly was true.

Another glaring dissimilarity between us concerned our jobs as student workers at the college cafeteria, which we had obtained as part of our financial aid package. From day one I loved working there and Deb hated it. Donned in gold jackets and brightly colored bandanas, we had to serve food directly to students as they passed through the line, and I think Deb felt self-conscious. I, on the other hand, was in my element — around food and, like an alcoholic working in a liquor store, I slipped comfortably into the job. The work was enjoyable, and I became efficient and good at what I did. I soon had a friendly rapport with both student and adult workers.

I was especially fond of my boss, Bert, and we developed a good working relationship. Under his management I found the joy that is possible when working for someone I both liked and respected. Bert was a hard-working man and always coming up with ideas to make eating and working at the cafeteria more pleasant and fun. Such things as letting students make their own sundaes on Sundays and having theme nights complete with specialty foods, decorations, and music.

I took pride in my work and did my best. Bert appreciated my enthu-siasm and gave me the responsibility of extra jobs. In all the times since my years with Bert, I have yet to work for anyone I thought more highly of.

As with previous employment, I was always on the lookout for chances to indulge my need for food. It was a standing rule that workers could not eat while serving, but in between rushes of students we all snacked frequently from the dessert selections. During noontime it was like working in a bakery with the cooks constantly replenishing the cookies and cakes, and it was tempting for anyone—diabetic or not. I routinely ate six to eight desserts and then smuggled one or two cookies back to the dorm. Most kids did take sweets out of the cafeteria, so I had no guilt about that.

By volunteering to come in early to set up the line or by staying late to clean up, I could get lots of extra eating in. I was also a willing substi-tute and thus earned bigger paychecks than anyone. I much preferred to work and the few times I ate in the dining hall, I was terribly self-conscious about going back for second helpings.

I made sure I was available to work any reception or banquet. It wasn't just the extra food or money—it felt good to be appreciated for my efforts. I felt more secure in the cafeteria than anywhere else on campus.

Bert and the other adult workers knew I was diabetic. I was never uncomfortable around Bert because he did not reprimand or embarrass me. Occasionally, he would quietly remind me that there was artificially sweetened fruit in the storeroom and I could help myself. But I never did eat any of it, refusing to admit that it would have been better for me.

There was only one person at the cafeteria whom I felt uneasy around, the woman who made salads. I did like her and in many ways she reminded me of my grandmother with her plump frame, white hair, and glasses. She'd remark often about my diabetes and, like my grandma, never raised her voice. Instead, she would put her arm around me and whisper softly that I should not be eating sweets. It was rather like nag-ging, but in a nice sort of way. At other times she would just look at me and I would feel guilty. I knew she must have eyes in the back of her head the way she always looked up just when I was reaching for some-thing to eat. I sighed with relief when her shift was over. Her good inten-tions only encouraged more devious behavior from me.

In contrast, I enjoyed getting to personally know the other cooks. We talked about many subjects, even my diabetes, but because they did not hassle me, I had no reason to avoid them.

As the first months of college flew by, home seemed millions of miles away to Deb and me for we truly loved our new world. Our grades were good and we were having the time of our lives involving ourselves in campus activities.

I had satisfactorily adapted my eating, drinking, and bathroom habits to my new environment. I was also illuminated with love and, although I did not get to spend much time with my boyfriend, Bob, because of his busy schedule as a music major, my infatuation with him kept me happy and hopeful. Bob was the only one who could tell me to take care of myself and it didn't bother me.

The last two weeks of the semester were more hectic than all the others. I kept extremely erratic hours studying for finals, finishing up term papers, and participating in holiday events. I felt a little run down but the excitement in the air kept me from thinking about it.

Deb and I would be driving home for Christmas vacation with our friends from church, Jon and Susan. The trip would be the beginning of a series of events that would not only endanger my life but widen the gap between my sister and me even further.

Chapter Eight

THE PRICE OF FREEDOM

THE FIRST TIME home from college is probably the most exciting in the four year experience, especially for kids like Deb and me who lived so far from home and only made it back for Christmas and summer vacation. We would have preferred to have flown from Nebraska and stepped dramatically off the plane, but instead, Jon, Susan, Deb, and I, and all our luggage were packed into a Volkswagen bug. We departed at 4 A.M. the day after classes ended. This was not a wise move for me, but I had not yet learned the danger of radical changes in my sleeping pattern. The nonstop trip was 21 hours long and the others were anxious to make good time, since there was ice and snow to contend with during part of the journey. I thought it exciting to leave in the quiet darkness of early morning, but going without sleep was the last thing I needed to top off the preceding busy weeks. Also, I had forgotten about not being able to go to the bathroom every half hour as I was accustomed to. For 900 miles, that is what I thought about — going to the bathroom and getting something to drink. I made no connection that these were the same symptoms I had had seven years earlier when coming down with diabetes.

We only stopped at gas stations every two to three hours, and I was miserable as my mouth began to feel parched and dry. I was afraid that if I let any of the others know how badly and how often I had to urinate I would be asked if I was okay, or Deb would accuse me for the millionth time of not taking care of myself. The fear carried me through to the next stop.

In anticipation of seeing my family I temporarily forgot my aching bladder as we drove the final few miles. As anticipated, our arrival was given the royal treatment and we were greeted like celebrities. Even Grandma had driven 150 miles to spend the holidays with us. It was to be a special Christmas for another reason. Mother was marrying Hank and there was much hub-bub over the wedding plans.

Christmas in our home always resulted in an abundance of sweets to which I fell victim. Grandma, who seldom did any baking, went all out at this time of year making and decorating several kinds of cookies. She brought the cookies to our house in two familiar looking canisters. She had used them for years for this purpose and I could spot them a mile away. One was blue with flowers and the other was white with a gold lid. This Christmas, as usual, I pretended not to notice them, but kept an eye out for where in the house Grandma shelved them. Then, during the night, or when no one was around, I would sample each variety. It was traditional for Grandma to write each family member's name on one of her coconut-oatmeal cookies. I was touched by the fact that even though I was reminded to stay out of the cookies, she always wrote my name on one of them too.

More alluring sweets appeared Christmas Eve when Mother received a large can of homemade fudge from my aunt. Everyone was offered a piece except for me, and my aunt made a point to say, "Those are not for you, Denny." I was aware that it was not for me. It never was, so why did my aunt have to embarrass me. I made no reply knowing that later I would help myself to the candy. It is sad that the only things I recall my aunt ever saying to me were to the same effect, "You have to take care of yourself," and "You can't have that."

Deb and I had such fun over the two weeks laughing and relating college anecdotes to our family and friends. Besides visiting and running around I spent considerable time eating, drinking ice tea, and going to the bathroom. With the thrill of being home and all the attention we were getting, I did not even think of my diabetes. However, I did mention to Mother that the trip home in the car had been rough on me. We talked it over and she said Deb and I could take a bus back to school. We found out that there was not a direct route and the ride would take 36 hours, but I did not mind because there was a restroom on the bus.

At the bus station when we left, it may have seemed like deja vu to an onlooker, but—unfortunately—none of us saw the similarity with the past. Mother told me I looked a little tired and she wanted to know if I was up to the long hours on the bus. I agreed to being a bit tired, but said I planned on sleeping most of the trip, and added that I would have an entire month to take it easy. January at our college was an interim month during which students could either enroll in a one-month long course, or take an extra long vacation. Mother, too, thought that sleep was what I needed after our whirlwind two weeks. Deb and I hugged and kissed Mother, Grandma, and Lisa good-bye, sad to leave but anxious to see our friends.

For the first couple hours of the trip Deb and I reminisced about the extra nice Christmas we had had and what fun it had been to compare notes with high school friends who attended schools of their own. I then tried to sleep but felt restless. Little did I know that these feelings of restlessness were but the tip of the iceberg. As the hours creeped by I became extremely dry-mouthed and nauseated. I couldn't figure out why I felt this way and assumed it was the lack of sleep combined with an upset stomach. I looked forward to our two-hour layover in Denver and planned to drink as much liquid as possible.

When we rolled into the bus stop, I rose from my seat and at once felt drained of all my energy. I had mentioned none of my discomforts to Deb, but now she noticed me holding onto the seats for support as we departed the bus. She was instantly worried and anxious, and she asked me what was wrong. I answered that I was very tired and thirsty and would appreciate it if she could first find me a restroom where I could sit while she got me something cold to drink.

She quickly led the way for me through a packed crowd of people. To my dismay, the lounge area had no chairs, couches, or even benches to sit on. My throat ached as I held back a sob and headed straight for a stall, where I collapsed onto a toilet seat to rest. Minutes later, I walked to the sink. Deb did not want to leave me but I insisted that I needed something cold to drink. She finally obliged and, in the meantime, I bent over the sink and gulped handfuls of water. After several gulps, a wave of nausea swept over me and I ran back to the toilet to vomit.

My mouth and throat were left foul-tasting and drier than ever so I returned to the sink for more water. Within seconds I was throwing up again. Now I was positive I must have the flu. I was too weak to stand any longer, so I sat on the floor, using the wall for support. Even this was too taxing and I leaned over to prop my elbow against the floor and lay my head in my hands. I had never felt this weak in my life.

Deb returned and was completely distraught to see me on the floor. She wanted to call Mother, but I insisted she not call and get Mother worried over nothing. Poor Deb was very embarrassed, and when two women walked into the restroom, she pleaded with me to get up off the floor. I was past the point of embarrassment. Though I was exhausted, sleep would not come. I sincerely thought I would be all right if I could just hold out till the end of the trip.

When Deb announced that it was time to reboard the bus, I was re-lieved that I would have a place to recline. My only memory of the next few hours is that they were agony for me as I tossed-and-turned trying to find a comfortable position and hopefully doze.

At the next stop in Cheyenne, Wyoming, I knew I was not strong enough to get off the bus. I told Deb to go without me and once again implored her to get me a drink with ice in it. I closed my eyes to wait for her, oblivious to the passing of time.

I heard Deb's voice telling me to wake up. My eyes opened and I saw that she was handing me a small can of fruit juice. I burst into tears. A heavily sweetened fruit drink was the last thing I wanted, for it did not sound like it would quench my thirst at all. Deb was now frustrated and angry because she thought she was doing what I had requested. She snapped at me, "Denise, what *do* you want?"

I choked out that I just wanted something with ice in it because I was so thirsty. Obviously perturbed, she left the bus for a second time. Glancing around I spotted a row of three seats in the back with no arm rests in between. I got up and stumbled over to them and lay down. The bus driver appeared and asked me if I was all right. I said "yes" that I was just tired and wanted to lie down. He told me I would have to go back to my own seat. I fought back tears as I made my way back. Deb brought me a Coke then and I downed it in two gulps.

On the next leg of the trip, I faded in-and-out of consciousness. The only thing that kept me going was knowing that as soon as the trip was over, I could sleep as long as I wanted in my own comfortable bed. Oh, sleep . . .

The next thing I was conscious of was lying on my back and gasping for air. There were people all around, but they were not helping me. In-stead, they were pushing on my chest and making it harder for me to breathe. They kept asking me questions which I could not answer be-cause I was concentrating so hard on trying to breathe. I attempted making a noise to show them that I could not speak, but nothing came out. My chest hurt tremendously as I heaved up-and-down trying to fill my lungs with air. I was barely cognizant of needles being put into me and tape being wrapped around my arms. After what seemed an eter-nity, my breathing got easier and I fell asleep.

When I awoke, tears stung my eyes—there was no mistaking that I was in a hospital. I.V.'s were in both my arms and there was an unbear-able pressure on my bladder which made me think I could not keep from wetting the bed. My chest ached and my mouth was so dry it would not open. Someone walked in and I asked for my sister. An attentive nurse explained what was going on. She said I was in a hospital in North Platte, Nebraska and had been brought there the previous day, after becoming unconscious on the bus. My sister had gone to the bus driver and told him I was very sick. The driver asked if she wanted him to call for an ambulance. Deb started crying and said she didn't know what to do because her sister had diabetes. He told her not to worry — he knew what to do since his son was also diabetic.

Again I had missed all the dramatics. Two ambulance attendants had brought a stretcher onto the bus, tied me to it, and carried me off while people lined up outside looked on. This time Deb rode in the ambulance with me.

Upon hearing the story, I was ashamed and depressed. I had honestly believed I only needed rest and had no idea I was sick enough to come to the hospital. I feared Deb's reaction to being put through all this. The nurse told me Deb was staying at the apartment of one of the young nurses who worked at the hospital and she would be coming to see me. I was hurt that Deb was not there waiting for me to wake up.

A while later, a doctor stopped by my room to inquire how I was feeling. He asked me some questions about the preceding weeks and how my diabetes was going. I said I had felt fine and even admitted to eating some candy at Christmas. I asked him what had happened to me. His entire explanation was that my diabetes "had gotten out of control." I was so tired of that phrase and at the same time did not understand its implication. Silently I cursed myself — it must be because of all my overeating. By the end of the day I was already feeling close to normal again, but was told I would have to remain in the hospital a couple more days to make sure.

When Deb came to see me she stayed only a few minutes. She appeared relieved to know that I was all right, but I could tell she was uncomfortable visiting with me. She said that Mother had been distressed to hear about me and wanted me to phone her as soon as I got back to the college. From now on, we would travel only by plane.

I apologized to Deb for all the trouble. She told me I had scared her when she was unable to get a response from me, and she was just thankful the bus driver had been so understanding. Deb was getting restless to go. I asked her to do me a favor and call Bob. She reluctantly agreed and left with a quick good-bye.

The following day Deb showed up for an even shorter visit, but with a good word for me. She had phoned Bob who was very concerned about me and also had a message — "Tell Denise I love her." This brought the first smile to my face in a while, and even Deb seemed touched by his sentiment. She left then to meet some friends and I did not see her again until I was released.

Several times I inquired about Deb from the nurse she was staying with. It sounded like everyone was enjoying Deb and she was having a very sociable time, even dating one of the x-ray technicians.

At hearing this I felt a sting of jealousy toward those who shared Deb's time, but I couldn't blame Deb for having fun and making the best of the situation. It wasn't her fault I was in the hospital.

Time passed slowly giving me little else to do but accept the loneliness I deserved and to contemplate. I was not angry and I did not cry. I was just immensely sad. I was learning that Deb liked being around me even less when I was sick. Her absence shamed me, and I could not tell her how much I was hurting. I felt a longing for the days when we had been close. When all of this was over, I would never let it happen to me again.

I was discharged after a total of four days, and even though I was still sore from my ordeal in the emergency room, I was more totally revitalized than I had been in years. I was physically and mentally strong, and it was wonderful to be alive! Within an hour, Deb and I were once again on a bus and heading for our home away from home.

When the taxi pulled up in front of our beloved Augustine Hall, Deb and I flew inside. We had not anticipated such an exciting welcome, but several of the girls had heard of our adventure and were waiting in the foyer to greet us. They could see for themselves that we were doing great, and there was much hugging, laughing, and talking. They were all acting like little mothers, affectionately warning me that I had to take care of myself. I smiled appreciatively, but inside I cringed because now there would be more people on the lookout for me and what I did.

Over the next few days I had to put up with some gentle nagging from the girls, who all meant well, and I just agreed with everything they said to avoid arguments. But their watchfulness made me feel like I was being nudged back into my dual role — the part others approved of and the secret me who could do what I wanted when no one else was looking. Later, during the night, I would go down to the basement where the dorm refrigerator was located and sneak fudge and cookies out of the boxes which girls had brought back from Christmas vacation. It was all right to do this because I was well now and I believed I would never get sick again.

Here I had the chance to make amends to my body, but instead I took advantage of its ability to heal itself. College was giving me the freedom to learn, to grow, to experience, and to choose. I was choosing not to see what I was doing to myself. As far as my health was concerned, that freedom was coming with a high price.

Chapter Nine

SECOND-HAND LOOK

MY SOPHOMORE year at college brought encounters of a different nature. Over the summer, the administration had turned our happy home, "Augie," into a male dorm and, sadly, all of us girls made the move to the larger Beegle Hall. Deb and I each had new roommates and we lived in separate wings of the building. While I preferred concerts, working on plays, and visits to the coffeehouse, Deb's free time was filled with sorority and Greek activities, which provided her a strong sense of identity.

On the rare occasions when we did things together, Deb seemed hurried and uneasy. Unless she invited me, things like going to the Student Union or eating at the cafeteria with each other were unspoken taboos. If there was at least a third person with us, the situation was more tolerable for Deb because she did not have to focus her attention on me. I put no demands on her and I grew to accept that her need for me came when she was lonely or depressed. At least I could offer her comfort and understanding.

Meanwhile, I had other preoccupations to contend with. Living in a larger dorm gave me a lot of anonymity. The 40 girls with whom I lived so closely my first year were now spread out among 300 girls, and this I used to my advantage. Most mornings between 12 to 2 A.M. found me frequenting the candy and snack machines and buying up to 50 items a week, which I ate in private and quickly. I'd have insulin reactions at odd hours of the night and used them as excuses to eat two or three candy bars, instead of juice or pop. These liquids would have entered my bloodstream far more rapidly than fat-laden chocolate, but I was unaware of this and probably would not have wanted to know.

When I had entered college my intentions were to major in some line of social work, but certain events turned me in the direction of education, primarily special education. During the fall semester of my sophomore year, I was a reader for George, the only blind student on campus. He was well-known and well-liked. I had first met George the year before at a Sunday night function for freshmen held at a nearby church. He had entertained us with guitar music and his beautiful singing voice.

I think all the girls were charmed by him that night and I am sure his blindness had something to do with his charisma. The majority of us had never been around a person who could not see and George's self-assuredness and outgoingness were appealing. He had a friendliness that radiated about him, a soft attractive voice, and a sexy laugh. I lacked enough self assertiveness to introduce myself to him that night, and I decided to watch for another opportunity. The perfect chance came two months later. My boyfriend, Bob, took me to lunch one Sunday with a group of his fraternity brothers and, to my delight, George was among the group. I was introduced and again found myself attracted to him. He captivated me completely when he read the sesame seeds on his hamburger bun as if they were Braille dots and announced to us that they read, "Shit!"

A few weeks later George, Bob, and I decided to have dinner together. As we walked in the door of the fast food restaurant, a woman coming the opposite way wasn't paying attention and bumped into George. Bob yelled, "Can't you see he's blind?"

To my immature attitude, I thought him noble for speaking up, but at the same time I felt uncomfortable for George and the woman for being singled out. Actually, it was Bob's words that had created the embarrassing situation.

The more I was around George, the more I was intrigued by his handicap, which, for him, did not appear to be a handicap because he got around so well. There were so many questions I wanted to ask him, but I was reluctant about getting too personal. For the remainder of the year I continued to speak briefly whenever I saw him.

When George mentioned that he needed another reader, I volunteered and was anxious to get to know him better. George had a photographic memory and never asked me to repeat sentences. I was forever amazed by his powers of retention. After the reading sessions we would walk back to his dormitory and I—caught up in the role of the Good Samaritan—was proud to be seen with him. I had seen George walking with other students and so patterned myself after them, letting him hold onto one of my bent elbows as we walked. Although he always carried a cane, he did not use it while holding on to someone's elbow.

If there was an object obstructing his path, I was uneasy and did not know if I should warn him or let him discover it for himself. So, rather than ask him if he needed such information from me, I kept quiet. This silence led me to make a fool out of myself and put George in a dangerous position once when we were walking across a parking lot. Straight ahead in our path was a parked car and I knew he would run into it if I did not say or do something. But I was too intimidated by the situation to do or say anything and let him walk right into the car. Then I, acting as if it had been an oversight on my part, apologized profusely. Typical of George, he took the incident calmly and laughed reassuringly and cracked a joke. I was the one with the hang up and his humor bailed me out.

As George and I became better friends, he learned of my interest in special education. He approached me on the subject and asked me if I would like to spend the coming January at the school for the visually handicapped which he had attended when younger. The school was in a small town about 200 miles from Midland. George told me he thought I would be sensitive to the children there. I was flattered that he thought to ask me and the idea sounded interesting. Arrangements were made between the school's superintendant, who George knew previously, and my advisor to make sure I would get credit for my time there. My advisor, who respected and admired George, thought it was an ideal opportunity and, in lieu of a test, I could write a term paper about my visit.

January rolled around and I was a bit scared to go out on my own, leaving behind my friends and the security of campus life. But I decided a month was not that long and if George had suggested it, it would be good. The night I arrived I was given a room in the girls' dorm.

The next day dispelled any doubts I may have had. The students I met were a combination of adorable, curious, and inspiring. About half of the students were totally blind and the other half had varying degrees of visual impairment. They were instructed to call me Miss Bradley. Over the next four weeks, I was allowed to sit in and/or participate in all classes and activities, and also to talk to each teacher individually. Each evening I wrote in a journal about my impressions of the day and what I had seen and learned.

The kindergarten and lower elementary classes were the most enjoyable for me partly because the younger ones opened up to me right away — they seemed fascinated by the presence of someone new — and partly because they were still learning the basics of getting around in a sightless world and were more interesting to observe. I loved to watch their tiny fingers read Braille and was amazed by one likeable little boy who wore very thick glasses and read with his nose pressed against the page of his book. The kids were like any other kids, their handicaps only being something unique about them like the color of their hair and the sizes of their bodies.

What the students of all ages did in their gym classes would have been hard to believe if I had not seen it for myself. They roller skated, swam, and bowled like experts. They skated forward, backward, and in figure eights, and stopped on a dime without running into a wall. The bowling lanes had old-fashioned pin-setting machines and each student had to take his turn at setting the pins — not an easy thing to do.

At meals, I was so absorbed in watching the children eat that I ate very little. I was impressed by their neatness and skills. Each child's place setting was treated like the face of a clock: drinking glass at one o'clock, silverware at three o'clock, and so on. They served themselves and passed around bowls as if they could see. I learned that it was all a matter of technique.

I learned to follow the children's example in their treatment of one another and became aware of how they used their other senses. The little kids especially showed no prejudice and were eager to help any of the others when able. The partially sighted kids would clap their hands so that the blind kids would know where they were standing. One little girl was black but this did not matter to any of them. I was drawn to a little blind girl named Denise, who was very intelligent and perceptive. She handled very confidently the role of leader which the other kids seemed to place her in. There was much touching and closeness between them.

Most of the kids had adjusted to life at the school and to being away from home. As in any school, there were a few outcasts and loners, but because they were blind they seemed more pathetic to me. Maybe I thought that way because that is the concept of a blind or handicapped person, that he is lonely. I was truly being confronted with a world I had never known, and I thought of maybe becoming a teacher for the blind.

Upon returning to Midland, I handed in my journal and after my advisor read it, he determined it so thorough that I did not have to write a paper. My diary of personal insights earned me an "A" for the course.

My time at the school had "opened my eyes" to many things I had come in contact with back on my campus. For one thing, handicaps seemed easier to deal with in small children than in older children or adults. Maybe I felt that I could rightfully help a child whereas there was an uncertainty in helping a grown-up person, like the way I had felt when walking with George.

My experience had at least taught me to be aware of other people, how they were different from, or like me. I thought ironically that a physical handicap was more honest and seemed easier to have because it was in the open for everyone to see and judge. I, too, in a sense had a handicap, but mine was hidden from others and I spent a great deal of time and energy keeping it that way.

Chapter Ten

WIN SOME, LOSE SOME

WITH MY two years experience of working in the college cafeteria, I decided to try waitressing for the summer of 1972, as a nice change of pace from working at the hamburger stand the previous year. I wrote letters of application to several restaurants in Albuquerque and heard from the manager of a Sambo's that I would be given an interview as soon as I got in town. I was hired that same day, and I was proud of myself for having sought out and got the job on my own.

My new boss asked me if I could work the graveyard shift and, as I enjoyed the late night hours, said "yes" right away. I was energetic and eager to become as good a worker as I was back at the cafeteria. Working the late shift proved to be very physically tiring. From nine at night to seven the next morning, I did not stop running. If I happened to get a short break, I'd grab a few crackers or a Coke.

I became friends with another waitress my own age and after our shift was over, we'd eat breakfast together. We were told we could eat any of the desserts, pancakes, salads, and even candy that we wanted. I mentioned to no one that I had diabetes. While the cook prepared our steak or eggs, we'd reward our hard work with huge sundaes and a few Hershey® bars.

I arrived home about 8 A.M. and then took my insulin. After a couple of hours of winding down, I went to bed, giving no thought to what effect the new schedule might have on my body or diabetes control.

About three weeks later I found out. Just when I was getting the routine down and increasing my tips, I began to feel listless and less enthusiastic about the job. Even a switch to part days and part nights did not help and was actually worse, because my sleeping pattern was now more irregular than ever. Mother made me quit, which would have been inevitable, for a week later I landed in the hospital. It was a relief to be able

71

to tell people that I was exhausted from working too hard. Even though the doctor told me that my body wasn't used to the new schedule and that I should have readjusted the times I took insulin and ate meals, I kept thinking that the real and only reason I was sick was from all the food.

The experience should have taught me that watching my food intake was not the only part of good control, that I needed to be aware of my routine and the importance of balancing eating, activities, and medication, but it did not. I was far from comprehending what living with diabetes was all about. My recovery back to normal only took two days and I was back at the hamburger stand and to my roller coaster existence within a week.

This brief stay in the hospital was nothing new to me. I had developed a pattern of going in about every six months. To me, these visits to my "second home" were only temporary interruptions of my freedom to do as I pleased.

The first time I was in the hospital in my college town reminded me of when I was 11 years old . . . constant visitors, gifts, and flowers. I kept telling everyone that I was not sick and it was just that my diabetes was out of control, using that phrase because it meant nothing to them. None of them understood diabetes or even bothered to ask me about it. Instead, they acted like I had the flu or something else I could recover from and return to normal. Maybe this was because when I was feeling good, I seemed as normal as anybody. How I had wished it had been that simple.

Whenever I was in the hospital, I was famished all the time and would daydream about food, thumbing through magazines for pictures of food to try and satisfy my hunger. I felt empty and deprived and also fantasized about escaping. Even after I was well the doctor would keep me in a couple of extra days to "keep me in control." But they were wrong, too, since my regular schedule was certainly different than my hospital one, and it was therefore an artificial type of control.

At this point in my life, there was less and less communication between me and the medical world. I did not have a regular doctor during college, and for minor ailments I went to the school nurse. When I was hospitalized, a doctor was assigned to me. Most of the doctors would never come to see me and just left orders with the nurse that I was not to be released until my blood sugar readings were lower. It burned me up—I had questions to ask and no one would tell me the results of my blood or urine tests, as if I had nothing to do with the control of my own disease.

I had a growing fear that not only did I know little about diabetes, but neither did the doctors have all or even most of the answers, and they did not like to be questioned about topics in which they were unknowledgeable. So I lay in bed thinking that the diabetes and the doctors were against me and felt lonelier than ever in my struggle.

On the other hand, as I did acquire some knowledge about diabetes just from the mere fact of living with it from day to day, the frustrations were still there. It was not rare for medical people to condescend to me. Over time, I realized that when I first began to throw up, it was a sign of "a point of no return." Although it would be years before I understood why I threw up, I did not know then that it meant I needed emergency care as soon as possible. When I reached this stage one time in the dorm, I initiated action and asked a friend, Noli, to drive me to the hospital. The emergency room was filled with people. I approached the admitting nurse, told her I was diabetic and what my symptoms were, and told her I needed to be put on a sodium I.V. immediately or I could go into a coma. I was breathing loud and forcibly and could barely stand up. She stared at me as if I was out of my mind and said that only a doctor could make a diagnosis or prescribe treatment. She said to take a seat and wait my turn. Before they located a doctor for me, it was a miserable hour, reminiscent of the infamous bus trip back from Albuquerque. I slumped in a chair, closed my eyes, and kept my mind concentrated on ice cubes, while poor Noli sat helplessly by. When the doctor finally got there, he put me on a sodium I.V. at once. I wished later that I had vomited in the nurse's face or passed out on the floor to get her to be attentive to my problem. I was bitter about the event for a long time.

Now I can see that because medical personnel — especially those in a hospital — always see diabetics at their worst, they take on the attitude that no diabetic knows what is best for himself.

I was now midway through my junior year of college. I thought it strange that girls began remarking about how skinny I was looking. Since I was so used to "feeling fat" and never looking at myself in a full length mirror that, at first, I laughed off their comments with an, "I *wish!*" But this "skinny" talk continued and finally I noticed that I did look smaller . . . could it be that my lifelong dream was coming *true?*

I decided to dig out an old two-piece bathing suit I had worn five months previous and had looked overweight in. When I slipped into the suit, I was shocked, for it fit comfortably and looked surprisingly good. I tried to think if I had been eating less than usual or if my weight loss could be attributed to my running up-and-down the stairs to my third floor room. Whatever the reason, I knew I had never dieted a day in my life, and — except for the times I was in the hospital — I ate like a football player.

The frequent comments continued and this type of recognition was a real boost to my self-esteem. Unfortunately, it was also an enabler to my food addiction. I was as hungry as ever, if not more so, these days. I began to eat large amounts of food in front of people and wasn't even embarrassed when they kidded me about it. The promise I had made to myself years ago about never overeating again if I could magically be thin was out the window.

As an explanation I started telling others that my metabolism had changed, which seemed reasonable to them and me, although in the back of my mind there was a gnawing little feeling that my unexplainable loss of weight might not be a good sign. I pushed the thought aside. It was a wonderful feeling not to be ashamed of my figure and to let my clothes show it off instead of just cover it up. I only wished that the other girls would tell me I had a good figure, like they always told Deb, rather than just saying I was skinny.

I kept my old clothes around to wear to work. One pair of jeans was way too big for me around the waist, so I had to wear a belt. I began to feel uncomfortable in them. My skin was tender and sensitive and I assumed it was the excess material causing friction. But then, even if I wore tighter jeans, the irritation persisted. When I took off the jeans there was a sort of stinging sensation around my hip area. I thought the coarse material was causing my soreness. I tried wearing tops which had to be tucked in and could serve as a lining between my skin and the jean material, but they didn't help much. Along with the sensitivity, my skin also itched. Luckily, the irritation was not constant and when it was not there I forgot all about it. I wanted to enjoy my new body.

The sensitivity continued to be annoying but tolerable for the rest of the semester. When summer came, Deb, a girlfriend, and I decided to stay in Fremont and get an apartment together instead of going home. The place we rented was a basement apartment which was very damp because of the high humidity and heat of the Midwest. My hips started bothering me again and I noticed my problem worsened when the humidity was high. I longed to be outside enjoying the sun, but if there was any moisture at all I couldn't take it.

Inside the apartment I kept the air conditioner running all the time, which made the air cold, but drier, and therefore more bearable. I wore my two-piece bathing suit almost exclusively while inside. Even the fabric of the couch and the sheets on my bed affected me, forcing me to sleep lying face down on a rubber mat to keep the sensitive areas of my body from touching anything. Eating helped keep my mind off my misery and I even took up smoking to divert attention from my body.

I had met a new friend, Len, who brought me much comic relief that summer. On humid days, when I was stuck inside, she would visit and entertain me with jokes and Elvis imitations. One hot sticky night after the lakes were closed, I wanted to go for a swim, because the cool water temporarily soothed my tormented body. Len suggested we drive around and maybe get into the pool at some motel. It was late and all the gates to the pools were locked, but I was in a daring mood so I jumped the fence at one place and went for a quick swim. Len waited in the car so we could make a fast get-a-way.

My summer job was as a cashier at a Walgreens store and female employees were required to wear nylons. For me, eight hours in panty hose was not only irritating but painful. One rainy day, I ended up in tears after walking the two miles to work; I had never itched so bad in my life. For ten minutes I violently raked my legs and hips with a hair brush, leaving them red and stinging. The itching was deep inside my skin and I wished for a sharp knife to dig it out. I was mad at my body for being so strange, at the weather for being so wet, at the boss for his stupid rule, and at myself for having diabetes. I could not go on with this wicked curse.

In July I quit my job rather than try and explain to the boss about my strange problem. To my dismay, the relief I had from not wearing nylons was short lived, and I reluctantly made an appointment to see a doctor. He was an older man who had treated me at the hospital and was a little more attentive to my problems than some doctors. I tried to explain to him the discomfort I had been having for so many months. I showed him that there was nothing to look at in the affected areas and expressed how the irritation seemed to come from inside my body, that it was mostly itching and burning, but sometimes felt like bugs crawling on my skin, or tingly feelings. He was puzzled and could only agree with me about the fabric or humidity causing the itching. Having a doctor not know what was wrong seemed worse than a negative diagnosis, and I began to wonder if it was all in my imagination.

I also told the doctor about my weight loss, and even added that I had not cut down on my eating, which was plenty. He asked me how I was feeling. I said the heat and humidity tired me, but I was fine except for the itching. Neither of us connected my weight loss with the problem in my skin and I figured I would have to accept this weird side effect as the price for being thin. I trusted the doctor and did not think to get a second opinion.

The next time I was home I consulted the doctor who had treated me during high school. No sooner had I described my dilemma than he was nodding affirmatively. He knew what I was referring to—it was a side effect of diabetes called neuropathy, and it had to do with damaged nerve endings. I should have asked what caused it, but all I wanted to know was if it would go away or get worse. His attitude and tone insinuated that neuropathy was another thing diabetics had to put up with and for the next several years I would believe just that.

At least knowing what I was suffering from made it easier to accept. The doctor gave me a prescription to help me sleep at night. Sleeping had become increasingly difficult as the very weight of the sheets on my skin kept me tossing and turning. The first few dosages were effective but wore off the longer I took them. This scared me because I had no desire to get into stronger drugs or become dependent on them. How was I to get a decent night's sleep?

Mother was sympathetic and made an effort to help me. We discovered that nylon or silk type fabric did not irritate my skin, and Mother bought me a long, lime-colored nylon lounger. It felt wonderful and I wore it whenever I was in the house. Mother had a new lightweight foam blanket which she had received for Christmas. It gave me such relief when I slept that she handed it right over to me and said I could keep it.

Back at school when it was damp in our unair-conditioned dorm even my nylon nightgown was uncomfortable. I tried wearing only underwear to bed, but then even the elastic waistband of my panties became too much to stand. I took the final step and slept in the nude, fearing only that there may be a panty raid which did happen every now and then. Actually I wouldn't have cared if the male raiders did take my panties as long as no one saw me naked.

My problem was eventually solved after Mother sent me beautiful gold satin sheets for my birthday. They felt heavenly against my bare skin and, even though I slid off the bed a couple of times, I began to sleep the night through. However, I had not seen the end of my skin problem by any means and it would get worse before it got better. Others continued to compliment my shape and I would smile and thank them. But secretly I wanted to slip out of my body and into anyone else's. I watched with envy the other students move freely about in their tight fitting clothes—an honored privilege I was not allowed. The joy I always thought I would have in being slender was disfigured by the reaction of my body.

Chapter Eleven

"I" TROUBLE

LESS THAN one year after my visit to the school for visually impaired children and almost paralleling the start of my skin problems, a series of events began which led to my losing part of something very precious to me. It all started innocently enough and I can remember that day so clearly. My girlfriend Sally and I were in my dorm room studying. I was reading a textbook and absentmindedly reached up to brush something away from my eye, thinking it a hair or a piece of lint or string. As I continued reading, whatever it was was there again. I brushed it away a second time, but the object stubbornly remained. "Darn it!" I said aloud.

Sally looked up from her reading and asked what was wrong. I said that something on or near my eye would not go away. She inspected my eyes and face but could not see anything. I insisted that something was in my eye when I tried to read. Sally picked up on the worried tone in my voice and, like she always did, made a comment to start me laughing. She calmed me by adding that tomorrow she would take me to an eye doctor she knew. We quit reading for the night and I put it all out of my mind.

The next day the doctor patiently listened to my confused account of the night before and then proceeded to examine my eyes. He explained that the object I saw was neither on nor near my eye, but inside it, probably a bit of blood in the vitreous humor, which is the jelly-like fluid filling the globe of the eye. Technically, nothing extraneous is supposed to be in this area because it will prevent light rays from reaching the retina. An obstruction is treated by the retina (viewing screen of the eye) as if it were an object outside the eye and in its field of vision. So I had actually seen the debris (called a floater), but not for the reason I thought I had.

His explanation fascinated me and I wanted to know what caused it to happen. He said people usually get a floater simply by straining their eyes as when coughing or throwing up, in which case it usually disappears. In my case, however, it might be caused by something else and he wanted me to see an ophthalmologist, who was better equipped to look into my eyes. I thought this doctor's concern to be genuine and agreed to see the specialist.

The ophthalmologist determined that the floater was due to the progression of my retinopathy, which another doctor had confirmed three years earlier when I was in high school. He said there was a type of surgery that could be done but I would require some recovery time. We decided I would have the operation done in Albuquerque, during January so I could rest at home for a few weeks.

Two months later Deb and I and a couple of girlfriends drove to Albuquerque for Christmas. I didn't let the knowledge of imminent surgery put a damper on my holiday spirit. After an exciting week, Deb and our friends returned to college, leaving me behind to have my first operation.

I faced this new experience with optimism and curiosity and was not afraid because I had no pain or severe vision problems.

My rapport with the surgeon, an ophthalmologist named Dr. Johnson, was exceptional. He was middle aged, had a fatherly countenance, and quickly put any anxieties I had to rest. He was the kindest, gentlest, and most open and honest doctor I have ever known. Realizing this was to be my first surgery of any kind, he was very patient and fully explained everything he did. He seemed to have a personal regard and respect for my eyes and for the human body in general. He was the first medical person to ever spark a desire in me to be healthy and take care of myself. Part of me wanted so much to confide in him about my problems with diabetes, but another part of me was afraid of disappointing him so I said nothing.

The operation I was having, photocoagulation, was uncomplicated and usually done on an outpatient basis, but because I had diabetes, I would spend one night there following the surgery.

The operating room was small and quite bare except for two stools and a machine about three-and-a-half feet tall. I was clothed in a surgical cap, gown, and slippers, and I was to be awake and sitting up for the procedure.

My eye was numbed with a shot, which was the only distasteful part, although having taken shots for years somewhat prepared me. It was like getting a shot in the gums from a dentist. My bottom lid was pulled down, and the needle inserted into the tissue surrounding the eye. I caught a glimpse of the long needle as it went in, but it was over so fast I had no time to be afraid. Next, a contact lens was fitted onto my eye to magnify the area in which the doctor would be working.

I sat at one end facing the machine with my chin resting on a small platform. Dr. Johnson sat facing me at the opposite end of the machine, and a nurse stood quietly by. Dr. Johnson gazed into a powerful microscope, which enabled him to see my retina in minute detail. He had to aim very carefully before firing each laser beam. As each zap sealed off another leaky blood vessel by burning its end, I would see a tiny flash of light and hear the machine click.

During the treatment, the ever kind, reassuring voice of Dr. Johnson was there. He carried on a one-sided conversation with me throughout, explaining what he was doing and what he needed me to do. My part was to hold very still, not talk, and to turn my eyes in whatever direction he instructed me. It was painless as he had promised. He also praised and encouraged me often, which not only uplifted me and kept fearful thoughts at bay, but also added to my confidence in him. It was all over in 20 minutes. He put a patch on my eye and told me to rest in my room, and he would visit me that evening.

My room was on a floor with other eye patients and it was nice to be treated like a normal person who had just had surgery rather than like a diabetic who was in trouble again. True to his word, Dr. Johnson came to my room to talk with Mother and me. He recapped the purpose of the surgery, which was not to right any wrongs, but to prevent any further wrongs. He also went over, until he was sure we understood, exactly what he had done to my eye and hopefully what would be the future for it.

Retinopathy, he explained, was a disease in which the blood vessels kept expanding into additional, unneeded capillaries. These new, minute vessels tend to be weak and when they bleed, the blood goes into the vitreous humor causing floaters like the one I had. The worst outcome would be if the entire vitreous filled with blood, resulting in total blindness. On the positive side, which was his prognosis for me, was that no more blood vessels would grow, and that the ones already there would remain sealed off. He admitted it was possible that I would have to have the treatment repeated, and the best thing to do was to keep a close watch on my eyes.

Dr. Johnson spoke with such compassion that Mother and I were full of certainty for only the best. Over the remainder of the month I had to take several kinds of eye drops, refrain from exercising and lifting and bending, and be checked by Dr. Johnson every couple of days. Toward the end of January, I got the go-ahead to return to school, with one restriction—to curb my exercising for a few months. This was no loss since I never exercised anyway.

Unfortunately, the bleeding did reoccur intermittently over the next year-and-a-half and I required more laser surgery on both my eyes. In between times I had new eye problems to contend with. One was that I began to have random pain in my eyes due to inflammations of the iris.

The first time this inflammation occurred, Deb, a friend, and I were spending a school break with our father in Kansas City. When I awoke one morning, one of my eyes was so sensitive to light that I not only had to keep my eyes closed, but also had to keep a blanket over my head to block out the least bit of light. Daddy got me in to see an ophthalmologist right away, and I was led into his office by my father. The doctor diagnosed my condition as "iritis," which was common in diabetics like me who were in the first stage of retinopathy. However, the iritis was not serious and could be cleared up with medication.

Of course, the doctor asked me the obligatory question, was I in control?, and I gave my usual half-hearted answer not really saying "yes" and not really saying "no." He, like so many other doctors, just rushed over this part of the visit and did not emphasize, much less mention, that good control could stop as well as prevent further damage and that I was suffering unnecessarily if I ignored my diabetes. Instead, I was again led to believe that progression of the disease was inevitable.

He gave me dilating drops to relieve the pain and antibiotic drops to stop the infection. The pain went away in hours and after several days the redness, too, and I dismissed the incident. Whenever the iritis reappeared, it did so suddenly and violently with no apparent cause. Now, I am certain that the flare-ups correlated with my high blood sugars.

After that first time, I knew relief was possible and I would get started on the eye drops at once. It seemed I was now using eye drops more often than not. Perhaps it was ill-fated that the pain could be stopped so easily, for I gave little thought, if any, to what harm these infections might be doing to my eyes. The only inconvenience was the temporary blurriness caused the dilation of my pupils.

Another problem was that my nearsightedness became more pronounced and I had to wear my glasses during class in order to see the blackboard. My eyes were also sensitive to sunlight and I donned sunglasses whenever outside. For close-up work I had to use a large, hand-held magnifying glass. In time, more floaters appeared and it became especially difficult to concentrate on printed material.

The new floaters resembled cobwebs or threads and seemed to swim across my line of vision. Actually, the floaters themselves did not move, but the gel in which they were suspended did as I moved my eyes from side to side.

Sometimes I would forget that the floaters were there and I would jump in surprise or instinctively bat at them. They gave me the creeps. The magnifying glass helped by forcing me to concentrate so I could focus. When my eyes were fixed, the floaters did not move and were undetectible. The concentration required was a tremendous strain and I tired easily. Little by little I reduced the amount of reading I did.

I had always wanted to take a drawing course and my chance came during my final semester of college. It was a big challenge, especially when the subject we were drawing was across the classroom, or several yards away when we were outside. I switched back-and-forth among sunglasses, distance glasses, and the magnifying glass. All this considered, I was surprised at how well I did and was pleased with my portfolio of accomplishments.

The damage taking place in my eyes was causing changes in my life, what I could do and how well I did it, but even this was not enough to change my behavior. Sadly, when it came to driving a car, I had little foresight and took it for granted that I would always be able to drive. Since most of us students did not have cars and either walked or got rides with others, I did not miss driving or think about it much. On the last occasion on which I drove a car I was unaware that it would be the final time behind the wheel for me. I always dealt with present situations and did not worry about the future.

My college career was coming to a close. The thought of leaving Midland and my friends was traumatic. College had given me the opportunity to dabble in new experiences and ponder later whether they had any moral, social, or personal value for me. With the status of a "student," I could proclaim to the world that I was preparing myself for it, while still being sheltered by the world of campus life. I did not want my senior year to end because it would be the first time that I did not have schooling to look forward to. Perhaps deep inside was also the realization that, because I had not solved many of my emotional or physical problems, I would have to take them with me.

Chapter Twelve

BREAKING AWAY

WITH GRADUATION behind me, I half-heartedly turned to face my future. Breaking away from this part of life that had so changed and enriched me was far more emotional than leaving home had been. With no specific goals in mind, I let events carry me along, gently easing myself into whatever lay ahead. My main objective was to be happy and feel secure.

The fact that it was summertime made the transition from student life to outside life an easier one. Also, I still had college ties. We girls who remained in Fremont continued to see each other, and because we were unable to find a place big enough for the three of us, Deb and her best friend moved into an apartment while I rented a room in one of the girls' dorms on the campus of which I was now an alumnus.

I kept busy with a job as a maid at a Holiday Inn, making the two mile trip to work on a bicycle I purchased with graduation gift money. Cleaning was always easy for me and I like working alone and being able to wear old, comfortable clothes. I figured I was getting exercise, too, because we were required to clean the rooms quickly and I did plenty of bending and stretching. The job did not pay much, but as long as I could afford room and board and had a little entertainment money, it was all right with me.

Deb's roommate, Rita, also worked at the hotel and it was nice to have someone around I knew. One day while on a lunch break, Rita remarked that she was used to cleaning human hair from her bathrooms, but this particular morning one of her tubs had been full of dog hairs and it had been quite a mess to clean up. I sympathized with her and said I was lucky because I never had hair in my tubs or sinks.

A few days later after I had been working there a total of three weeks, I was summoned to see the hotel manager. As I walked to his office, I felt neither scared nor nervous, just curious. He was friendly and told me that upon inspection, my rooms looked great except for one thing—hair had been frequently left in the sinks and tubs. I was shocked and embarrassed . . . and immediately it hit me that I had missed the hairs because I had not seen them. I explained to the manager that I did have vision problems, but I had honestly thought my bathrooms were spotless. Although he was understanding, he said he would have to let me go, but would give me an extra two weeks pay because I was not given prior notice. I respected him and knew he had been right to fire me. Losing the job didn't matter to me as much as the fact that my eyesight had worsened so slowly I had not noticed.

When I had just about used up the severance pay, a former classmate told me that a school in town was looking for someone with a teaching degree to help run a summer recreation program for trainable mentally handicapped children. The girl said she had been hired for the physical education part, but they still needed someone to supervise the arts and crafts. She said she would recommend me if I was interested. I definitely was. The school, called The Opportunity Center, was the place where I had done part of my student teaching and I was familiar with the children who went there. The interview was only a formality and I was hired to start with only two days to prepare.

The session lasted a month and was good experience for me. I directed different projects for the kids to work on according to their capabilities. In addition, I went along on the swimming trips three times a week.

During August great things happened for me. I moved to a furnished, two bedroom apartment, which was near the campus and half-a-block from the downtown area. I was thrilled to be within walking distance of stores, banks, and the post office.

It was now fall and I knew it was time to start looking for permanent work. When an acquaintance told me of a part-time job that was open at a residence for mentally handicapped children, I jumped at the chance. The situation sounded ideal—the house was a short bike ride from my apartment and the hours would likely increase to full time.

When the houseparents had reviewed my qualifications, I was offered a position as one of the Resident Assistants, and I accepted. The couple had also gone to Midland. The girl, Nita, had lived in the same dorm as I when we were freshmen, but she had dropped out of school to get married. I tried out the job for a week and loved it. Unlike teaching in public school, which entailed mountains of paperwork, this job was informal and required little reading or writing.

Working 20 hours a week gave me plenty of spare time. I was kind of lonely as I could not yet afford a phone, and Deb and our friends worked full time at their various jobs. The loneliness was tempered with my new freedom — freedom from the watchful eyes of others. For the first time in my life, I was able to eat whenever and in whatever quantities I wanted. But any joy wore off fast; I still felt devious and unable to control myself. I took up smoking again which was merely a food substitute, as was the gum I chewed constantly.

As to my eyes, I was slowly adjusting to my lessened vision. I kept my magnifying glass with me at all times. Reading appealed to me, but even with large print books it was a great strain on my eyes. But at least the magnification allowed me to easily read letters, bills, and labels.

What troubled me more than my vision was the neuropathy which was still present from my waist down. My feet were not itchy or sensitive, but had slight numbness, which was also supposedly common in diabetics. At night, in order to sleep, it was necessary for me to lie on my couch directly in front of the air conditioner. Along with the itching and tenderness, I now got frequent shooting pains and a restless feeling in my legs.

While walking home from a dentist appointment one day, I decided to run part of the way. Within minutes my legs heated up and the deep internal itch returned. I immediately slowed to a walk, but the feeling would not go away. By the time I reached my apartment, I was in tears and again took a brush to my legs. Frantic with anger and distress, I sobbed and cursed out loud. Then I lay face down on my bed and cried myself to sleep. When I awoke the itching had stopped, but I vowed I would not exercise again for a long time.

Aside from the skin irritation, I had felt vibrant and energetic since my last hospitalization the previous spring. After I had been at my job a month, I started to feel listless and tired. Resting over a three-day vacation did not help, and I thought maybe I should tell someone I was not well. It was unusual that neither Deb nor any of my friends had stopped by to see me for at least three days. Sooner or later I knew one of them was bound to drop in, and so I stayed in bed another day. I faded in and out of sleep and could feel the last bit of strength draining out of me as the minutes ticked by. Still no one came and by that time I was too weak to even attempt getting down the steep stairs outside my front door to use my landlady's phone. There was no handrail and I was afraid that I would collapse and hurt myself. Yelling down the stairwell would not have helped since my 90-year-old landlady was almost totally deaf.

When the extreme thirst and vomiting began, I knew it was the same old thing—my diabetes was out of control. Slowly I would drag myself to the kitchen just long enough to make and inhale a pitcher of instant ice tea, then barely make it back to bed before passing out. Ten minutes later I would rush to the bathroom to throw up the tea. There was no doubt in my mind that I had to get to a hospital, but I was trapped in my upstairs apartment.

I began to worry and cry about the mess I had gotten myself into. At least all the other times, people were within reach to help me. Now, my life was not in my own hands and I had no idea what to do. I sobbed beseechingly.

For I don't know how long I lay there in agony and breathing heavily. All at once I was startled from my daze by the sound of someone hollering up the stairs. From my bed I yelled back, anxious to know who it was. I tried telling the stranger that I was too sick to come to the door. My voice had such little volume I was scared to death I would miss my only chance to be rescued, so I just moaned out loud.

Then I heard footsteps creaking on the stairs and I breathed a prayer of thanks. Luckily I had left the door unlocked, and I was never so happy as when I saw a figure appear at the doorway of my bedroom. I was very surprised to see that it was Mrs. Gigstad, the mother of one of my college friends, Karleen, who had lived in the apartment previously to me. She said she stopped by to see if her daughter had left anything behind. She could tell I was sick and asked what she could do to help. I implored her to call my doctor and find out if he wanted me to go to the emergency room. I told her what my symptoms were and she hurried out to make the call. A few minutes later she returned with orders to go to the hospital at once.

I sat up in bed and put on a pair of sandals that were lying nearby, while Mrs. Gigstad grabbed the nearest jacket she could find, a red-and-white plaid one. She helped slip it over my lime green nightgown, neither of us wondering about or caring how outlandish I must have looked. She supported my weight with her arms around me and we somehow managed to get down the stairs. I put all my concentration into walking as I feared each step would be my last before my legs would buckle underneath me. But they held out to her car and from her car to the hospital.

As I lay on the emergency room table, I said goodbye to Mrs. Gigstad and told her she had probably saved my life and I was grateful. She said she was glad she stopped and hoped I would be okay.

An I.V. needle was put into my arm and I relaxed because I knew that soon I would be all right. The I.V., by bypassing the stomach, restored lost body fluids and stopped the process of dehydration. Extra insulin lowered my blood sugar and within hours my body began to feel normal again. My stay was a short one, four days. I was anxious to get back to work. Deb drove me home. She felt bad about not having stopped by my apartment and promised to check regularly with me.

My ordeal over, I was prompted to get a telephone installed in my apartment but I was turned down because I only worked part-time and I didn't have money for a deposit. It was essential that I get one and I again felt victimized by my diabetes. Not knowing what else to do, I wrote Mother. It was hard asking her for money, something I hadn't done in years. Mother forwarded a check right away.

Back at the residence my weekly hours were increased to include five more hours with the kids and fifteen hours of housecleaning. The houseparents were aware of my vision problem, and yet they trusted that I would do a good job. Cleaning the large, three-story house and washing five loads of laundry daily kept me moving and made me feel better too. I adored the kids and became friends with all the workers, which gave me a sense of security. We shared a family-type togetherness and I knew, finally, that I had a happy, fulfilling world that did not include my twin or her reaction to my diabetes.

The nature of my work—one-to-one contact—was challenging as well as fun. I was learning to empathize with handicapped children, maybe because I too had a handicap and did not feel uncomfortable around them. I liked teaching the kids daily living skills, exercising them, or just playing with them. The only duty I did not perform was driving. Also, I felt more at ease with the kids who could not walk or who walked slowly because I could better keep an eye on them. It was after one little boy, Danny, slipped out of the house without me noticing, that I faced the reality of my visual limitations. Luckily, the other staff members located Danny, unharmed, and wandering the streets a few blocks away. They understood and were not angry with me. I liked that they had a respectful attitude toward me, ready to help when necessary, but never condescending or patronizing.

Nita, the housemother, had a delightful relationship with the children. She was so accepting of their handicaps, but at the same time could joke about them in a loving and understanding way. Whenever I took the little deaf boy, Jimmy, for a walk we'd laugh because he always dragged along in protest. Nita said it was "the blind leading the deaf!" I found her attitude refreshing and natural, and I followed her example.

None of us ever pitied the kids, but were drawn closer to them by having a sense of humor about their problems and appreciating their individual attributes.

For Christmas neither Deb nor I would be going home, but I did not mind because there was much holiday spirit and bustle in the air at the residence. A giant tree had been put up and the staff was planning a big party to be held a few nights before Christmas Eve. On the day of the party, the excitement heightened around the house — even the kids felt it.

One of them was Brian, a charming boy of 13, who had a mental age of about three years. He was understandably jealous of the younger or smaller children who could do things he could not because of his large size. We played with him on the floor or ran outside with him to help make up for some of the things he missed. Sometimes he got a little rough in his enthusiasm.

On the afternoon of the party I was holding Jimmy in my arms swinging him back and forth in a playful way. Out of the corner of my eye, I saw Brian smiling and running toward us, but my reaction time was slow and he charged into us. Jimmy and I fell hard against the carpet and my ankle was violently twisted. Other than being a bit dazed when I sat up, I felt fine and turned to check on Jimmy. He was weeping silently, but seemed to be okay. As I began to stand up, I collapsed on the floor and at once my foot tingled all over. I was carried to the couch and my ankle inspected. It had started to swell but did not hurt much . . . it just felt numb. Nita rushed me to the hospital for an x-ray. An x-ray technician told me there were no broken bones and that I had probably sprained a muscle.

I decided to go home and elevate my foot for a few hours in hopes of returning for the staff party. My foot continued to be swollen, but it did not hurt, and I took that as a sign that the injury was not that bad. With my foot wrapped in an Ace® bandage, I went to the party and walked and danced all night. This was the worst thing I could have done, for the next day my foot was red and puffy. I was forced to stay off it for several days, and only getting up for eating, going to the bathroom, and taking insulin shots.

When no change had occurred, I went to see the only doctor in town I was familiar with (the one who had not known what neuropathy was). He advised me to stay off my foot a while longer, adding that I could walk some if my foot did not hurt.

After a week the swelling remained but there was no pain and I was weary of sitting all day. I told Nita I would resume my cleaning duties and just see how it went. The difficult part was going up-and-down the stairs which caused shooting pains in my calf. I walked slowly and with a limp but figured that as the muscle healed, walking was good to get it back into shape. After many days the swelling started going away, and I thought I had done the right thing in returning to work. However, where the swelling had been, there was now a hard lump on the upper left side of my arch. This lump puzzled me for I could not figure out what it was. One day a friend of mine who was a physical education major urged me to see the doctor again and even hinted that I may have to wear some sort of brace to support my foot.

Her words were alarming and sounded a bit far-fetched, but I decided to be safe rather than sorry and went back to the doctor. He was as perplexed about the situation as I was. He recommended that I see an orthopedic specialist in Omaha. If only this advice had come a month earlier.

The specialist, along with several other doctors, x-rayed and examined my foot and asked a lot of questions. Then the specialist called me into his office. I limped in and sat down. He gently took my injured right foot in his hands and caressed it while he talked. In a concerned voice, he explained that the nerve damage in my feet from the diabetes had caused me to lose some normal sensations such as pain. When I sprained my foot, the relative lack of pain encouraged me to walk, whereas a person with a normal foot never would have been able to do so because of the intense pain. The sprain left the tendons and cartilage in a weakened state, and my continuous walking had put excess pressure on the bones which, in turn, began to move out of their natural position. Thus the hard lump on my arch was actually a dislocated bone.

This news stunned me. I asked if anything could be done for my foot. He said yes, that there had been a new type of brace developed for my kind of injury, and having one made would be the best thing for my foot. Imprints of my foot wouldhave to be taken so that a properly fitting mold could be made. As he talked, my girlfriend's prophecy rang through my mind.

Later I was angry. I felt betrayed by doctors who had never really explained the nature of diabetic foot complications. My feet had been examined numerous times in the past. The doctors always asked if my feet had any numbness and I always answered yes. The only response from them had been a nod of the head, again just agreeing that diabetics could expect this to happen, and I went on thinking that that was all it was — a funny feeling in my feet. Their fallacy was in not telling me what the ramifications of numbness were, that because of it, I may not be able to correctly interpret the occurrence of seriousness of injuries because I would either not feel the pain, or the pain would be minute, or the pain sensations I did have would be distorted. It should have been stressed that I needed to be extra cautious of any foot injury and not to compare myself with people who did not have diabetes, and, most of all, that I should no let the lack of pain be considered a good sign. As usual, lack of communication seemed to be the culprit.

Within two weeks I was wearing my new brace along with orthopedic shoes. The brace was made of a skin-colored, lightweight plastic material. It fit under my foot and up the back of my calf, beginning just under my arch and ending just under the back of my knee. There was a heavy Velcro® strap at the top and I also wore a sock to help keep it in place. It was more comfortable to walk with a limp because the brace kept my toes from properly bending. At first I was self-conscious inthe orthopedic shoes because the right one was larger to accommodate the brace, but with jeans on, they looked much like the fashion of the day.

I routinely visited the specialist in Omaha so he could keep watch over my foot. On one visit it came out in conversation that the brace would never correct the original damage, and that it was serving more as a protective measure to prevent the same thing from happening again. I was very upset at hearing this but said nothing to the doctor, because he had been so kind and concerned. I had believed all along that my foot would eventually heal, and again I felt deceived. Inside, a wave of distress was growing toward the very people who were supposed to be helping me.

In time I became accustomed to the brace and accepted the interruption it caused in my life. On the inside, my body was not in the best of shape, but outwardly I still had a slender figure, I could still walk, I could still see well enough to get around on my own, and I was emotionally happy with my job and my social life. I would take in stride whatever came my way.

Chapter Thirteen

THE BEST MEDICINE

THE ATTITUDE I had developed toward the handicapped children I worked with — that of seeing beyond and finding the humor in limitations — began to spread to other areas of my life. I was learning to look at the lighter side of the physical challenges I faced. Humor, I believe, was always within me, but surfaced at this time because I was most in need of it. I love laughing and the way it has of making cares and worries temporarily nonexistent, and laughing at myself taught me not to take life so seriously.

It was fun referring to myself as Sherlock Holmes with my magnifying glass, or to joke about the "dainty size" of my large orthopedic shoes.

The results of this attitude were entirely positive, serving not only as a diversion from my body but also as an avenue of acceptance for others. When I displayed a sense of humor showing that I was not sensitive about my handicap, those around me were more at ease. Being called "batty" because I was "blind as a bat" was funny when I knew the person saying it was laughing with me and not at me.

At work I felt the most comfortable because we all laughed at abnormal situations anyway. I remember that when we took the kids to a public place, humor was about the only way to survive the stares and aura of embarrassment that people directed toward us. After all, when you have a group of kids who are either drooling, making funny noises, or trying to shake hands with total strangers, you can't just ignore them. Others often saw the kids only as different and odd, but by our seeing something funny in what they did, we staff were really made aware of how normal the kids were in their need for attention and love, and to learn about their world and how to function in it.

Danny, for example, was fascinated by anything that was long and dangled, such as curtain cords, ropes, and shoelaces. Once at a J.C.

Penney jewelry counter we stopped him just in time from ripping down a display of necklaces. His ability to seek out and even invent things to dangle was amazing. He could shred a single sheet of paper toweling into a skinny, three-foot-long "dangle." Nita said that Danny had invented the "theory of dangletivity!"

These days I was feeling a new sense of power over my problems. It was during this metamorphic period that I met Steve, whose love and friendship would add many dimensions to my life. The organization of the residence had changed and we no longer had live-in houseparents. We all worked different shifts and only the children lived there full time. Steve was hired as one of the overnight staff to come in at 9 P.M. and stay until after the kids left for school the next morning.

The first thing I ever heard Steve say made me chuckle out loud. Some of us at work were kidding Steve about him never getting any sleep because of his overnight job. Steve answered us very matter-of-factly, "What is sleep, but little chunks of death." There was a moment's pause, then we all started laughing. From that moment on, I zeroed in on his low-key, dry sense of humor, finding it delightful.

I looked forward to the mornings when I was assigned to help Steve get the kids ready for school because I knew they would be enjoyable and full of laughs. Steve fit right in with the way the rest of us felt about the kids. He respected each child's intelligence and treated each as an individual. He had a good rapport with all of them. In addition, he was thorough in his work and calm in a crisis and always there were his underlying humorous observations about it all.

As we became friends, Steve noticed that I frequently joked about my vision and he asked me what was wrong with my eyes. It was so unusual for anyone, especially a male, to be so direct, and I liked that. Except for my eating compulsion — still going strong — I was upfront with him from the start, telling him about my diabetes and eyes and foot problems, and he showed sincere interest. The special combination he possessed of intelligence, compassion, and wit was very appealing to me.

On one of my off days from the residence, I scheduled a rare visit to the doctor. My blood was tested and I was told that my blood sugar was quite high. The doctor suggested that I test my urine for sugar once in a while and if there were large amounts, take five extra units of insulin. He said this might keep me from ending up in the hospital every six months. I had never heard of taking an extra dose of insulin beyond my prescribed amount, but I liked the idea. I continued my usual eating and the extra insulin must have helped because I felt pretty good.

When I returned to the doctor's a couple of weeks later, to my surprise my blood sugar reading was just as high as before. I felt so good, but the doctor was concerned. He then did the best thing he had ever done for me. He advised me to check into the university hospital in Omaha which had a Diabetes Clinic, where I could get a refresher course on the basics of diabetes. Later I would think that he should have taken his own advice. It was only after meeting the staff who ran the clinic and being impressed by them, that I agreed to be admitted for ten days.

Having never been in a university hospital before, I was surprised by the constant procession of student doctors into my room each day. All of a sudden the head doctor and six or eight of his curious disciples would surround my bed and the curtain would be drawn, adding drama to it all. The outgoing head doctor, with his red hair and checkered suit jacket, gave me the impression he was showing me off as a visible, true-life example of what the textbooks described.

The attentive students were encouraged to look into my eyes, examine my legs and feet, and test my slow and/or abnormal reflexes. I tried to joke with the doctors but they remained serious. The students stared at me with stoic expressions as their leader spouted off strings of medical terms. I didn't know whether to feel humbled, or courageous for being able to survive my "grave condition." Again, the emphasis seemed to be on what diabetes could do to the body, not why side effects occurred or how they could possibly be prevented.

Ironically, the education part of the program at the Diabetes Clinic was better than I had expected. I learned about insulin and the way it reacts in the body, why I got reactions, why urine testing was important, and—most critically—how to plan a schedule around me rather than around the diabetes.

Also for the first time since getting diabetes, I was given a definition of "blood sugar" I could understand. Prior to this the term had never quite jelled in my mind. All I had learned about blood sugar was that mine was never right, and that this vague entity, somewhere in my body, seemed to have a power all its own. And the numbers sometimes used with the term blood sugar meant nothing to me.

Whereas previously I had believed that blood sugar was something I should not have, now I learned that we all must have a certain amount of sugar (glucose) in our blood at all times, as it is the main source of energy for our cells. In diabetics the trick is to keep the blood sugar from raising too high or dropping too low. Upon learning this, I thought how simply it could have been explained if someone would have reversed the words and said that diabetes is controlled by controlling the amount of "sugar-in-the-blood."

To think that ten years had gone by from the time I acquired diabetes to the time I understood the most crucial and elementary term — blood sugar. It's difficult to deal with a problem if you don't understand it.

I was introduced to a relatively new method of testing for sugar in the blood that was due to revolutionize the way diabetics control their diabetes. The way I found out my blood sugar level was to go to a lab, have blood drawn, and wait several hours for the test results. But now there was a test an individual could do at home in just a few minutes. The method was similar to the test I was supposed to be using to monitor the amount of sugar in my urine. A single drop of blood was put on a strip of paper that had been chemically treated so that it would react to the sugar in the blood. The strip would then change color, and this color was compared to colors on a chart. Each color stood for a different level of sugar in the blood.

Or, instead of using the color chart, the strip could be placed into a meter which "read" the strip. An arrow on a screen would point to a number which indicated the amount of sugar in the blood. The meter was especially helpful as it was hard for me to distinguish between the different colors of the chart with my poor vision. It was suggested I might want to purchase a meter and start regularly testing my blood. The price of the machine was $1,000 and this was not covered by insurance. It was because of the high cost and my nervousness at lancing my fingertip for blood, that I decided not to buy one of the meters. Later my decision would haunt me.

One area which was only skimmed over was that of side effects. In a filmstrip I was shown, the usual statistics were given regarding blindness and amputation, but there was no mention that these conditions could develop over a long period of time, and I did not acquaint my present problems of eye infections or skin sensitivity with them.

Steve was there to pick me up after my release from the hospital. Right away he told me how healthy I looked. Happily, I expressed how I had learned so many things I'd never known before, that I was actually excited about putting all the facts of diabetes to work in my life. I even made a commitment to regularly test my urine. Over the next month I was successful at keeping test results and following a diet. I felt good and believed my efforts were paying off.

In the fall of that year, Steve and I moved in together. My family, including Deb, was shocked. They condoned this action only because they thought Steve could take care of me. After all I was a poor, sickly, diabetic with failing eyesight, and so moral judgments were overlooked. But not having my family's blessing did not bother me. Steve and I were in love and happy and felt right about our decision — that was all that mattered.

I had discussed birth control with the doctors at the Diabetes Clinic. The consensus was that all methods were risky, either because of the rate of effectiveness or of the increased rate of infection. The pill was popular with girls my age, but I was told that it was not a wise choice for diabetics, as there had not yet been enough studies carried out.

I was directed to see a gynecologist and we had a long, intimate discussion. We talked about my lifestyle and my plans for the future. He told me that if I sincerely wanted a baby, he would get me through the pregnancy, but he could not guarantee what it might do to my health. Besides the importance of keeping the blood sugar in control, the strain of labor could have serious effects on the blood vessels in my eyes. I weighed the pros and cons of temporary versus permanent methods and the risk to my body should I ever decide or accidently become pregnant. I determined a tubal ligation would be the best for me. This is a simple operation in which the ends of the Fallopian tubes are cauterized. It is irreversible and permanent.

The doctor, however, would not let me make such an abrupt decision, and I respected him for this. He said I was to consider it for at least two weeks before he would operate. The waiting period did not change my mind. Steve said the decision was mine to make. I felt that the chance of infection from an I.U.D. or any of the other temporary methods was the last thing I needed. The desire to maintain my own health, for what it was, seemed to override any debate about having children. Also, I secretly dreaded the thought of having to stay in strict control and under the constant watch of doctors for nine months. My mind was made up.

The operation was ordinarily done during an office visit, but I was required to stay two days in the hospital "just to make sure." All went smoothly with no pain or regrets.

In retrospect, considering my health at the time, I still think I made the best choice. Were I able to have a baby now, I fully trust that today's technology would allow a healthy pregnancy with no ill effects to my health. The important thing is that I, or any other diabetic woman who wants to have a baby, would have to be highly motivated and willing to make strict control of diabetes the primary objective. Once in a while I get a pang of motherhood or self perpetuation and realize that I will never know the experience of pregnancy or giving birth, but at these times, I only contemplate and do not regret the past.

Steve and I had been together a little over a month when my bubble of happiness burst apart. First the itching and sensitivity in my waist, hips, and legs increased to a level I could barely tolerate. Then my face broke out in the worst acne I had ever had. I suffered from insomnia and problems with elimination. I went back to the Diabetes Clinic and was given medication for each of my symptoms. What baffled me was that for the first time in a decade I was doing all the "right" things. What was going wrong?

For the next several weeks my health continued to spiral downward and along with it my mental attitude. I began to have pain in my stomach area, which can only be described as a block of cement being lodged there. All I wanted to do was curl up in a fetal position and lie still, as the pain was so constant and consuming that any movement made me more aware of it. Although concentrated in my stomach, the pain seemed to radiate outward and I was sensitive everywhere.

My once ravenous appetite was totally gone. Not eating is just as bad for a diabetic as overeating, and Steve, being aware of this, would make food for me and patiently coax me to eat a few bites. Even drinking was painful and I could only take a tiny sip at a time. It seemed like years, not just weeks ago, that I had so easily consumed large amounts of food and liquid.

At work, time went slowly and I moved like a zombie and hated the feeling of clothes against my body. I would roll up my blouses and tops to bare my stomach area and leave my jeans unfastened to relieve the friction of fabric to my waist. The staff understood my problem and did not seem to mind how I looked, but when a new manager came in, she told me I did not look professional or proper and to please cover up. She was right, but that did not change my condition. I started wearing Steve's old shirts which hung down far enough to hide my exposed skin.

I patiently waited for my work shift to end so that I could go home, put on a bikini, and not think about anything. The weather was now very cold and I would turn up the heat in our apartment to 90 degrees and poor Steve sweated profusely while I tried to keep warm. On the nights I was unable to sleep, I sat in our living room, smoked cigarettes, listened to records, and fantasized about dying. Never had I had such thoughts, but death seemed like a welcome relief from it all.

Two more agonizing weeks and I returned to the clinic to meet with the doctors. While trying to explain the stomach pains to them, I started crying because just the effort of talking hurt so much. They told me what I dreaded to hear — all they could figure out was that the pain probably came from neuropathy of my internal organs and nothing could be given for it except pain pills. The prognosis was that probably the pain would eventually go away. Hearing this crushed my spirit. Why couldn't the pain be caused by a tumor so that it could be cut out or treated. I hated the strange "nerve" explanation and that it all came from the diabetes. What was the use of staying in control if I had to suffer anyway because I had already ruined my body?

The only diversion from my depression was Steve. It wasn't his patience, understanding, gentleness, love, or optimism that helped me the most, although he gave them all. It was his dry, natural humor which he did not try to stifle. When I felt miserable, he would tease me about wearing a bikini in the wintertime or ask me, "Can I touch your hair or does that hurt too?" Others in my situation might have been turned off at this lack of seriousness, but when it was the last thing I felt like doing, he would make me laugh. He used perfect psychology with me to get my mind off my body and the pain.

Just when I thought I could take no more distress, more came. The floaters which had originally appeared in my eyes were small, and they were not always noticeable because of their location in my side vision. I had become used to them. One November morning I woke up and was sitting in bed. I could not see very well and blinked my eyes a couple of times to make sure I was awake. Everything was very dark. Holding my breath, I glanced from side-to-side . . . then I let out an anguished cry, for what I saw were large, black stringy masses right in the middle of both eyes. I felt lonely and frightened and called out for Steve. He was beside me in a second and tried to calm my sobbing body. I choked out what was wrong and told him I just knew that they were more floaters. I do not remember ever being more scared than I was in those few moments. Steve said we would see the eye doctor that day.

I went into the bathroom to fill my insulin syringe like I did every morning. I looked at the syringe barrel to see if I could read the numbers. I could not and that brought on a new rush of tears and swearing. Steve filled the syringe for me and talked quietly, sensing that humor was not appropriate that morning.

It was hard to concentrate on anything, so I just dressed, sat down, and waited for the doctor's office to open. The thought kept going through my mind that this could not be happening to me. I closed my eyes and fixed them into a stare so that I could not see the floaters that were swimming inside my eyes.

A short while later I felt less stressful when Dr. Waring (who had diagnosed my first floater) walked into the examining room. He was always straightforward and kind. He told me that although it was blood I was seeing, my blood vessels did not appear to be bleeding at present. He said there was a possibility the floaters would be reabsorbed into my body, but he could not say how long that would take if it occurred at all. He knew that by now I had had three laser surgeries on my eyes, but he said that more was not indicated. He told me to see an ophthalmologist in a month.

His words gave me some hope and I tried to be optimistic, but I felt so limited and just wanted it all to go away. Riding my bike was now impossible and I wondered if I would be able to work. What in the world was I going to do?

At work everyone was supportive and did my part of the paperwork while I played with the kids. As the days went by I realized that my initial fear was gradually dissolving. I decided to take one situation at a time and not push myself into frustration. I even felt a stirring of hope that things would actually turn out okay.

Steve got an unexpected phone call from a college friend offering him a job. The position, editor at a weekly newspaper, was open immediately. Steve asked the caller to hold a moment while he asked me if I would like to move to Phoenix, Arizona. I sat itching and shivering in my bathing suit, and feeling restless. Outside snow was falling. The thought of moving to a hot, dry climate sounded like heaven, and I gave him a resounding "Yes!"

Within days Steve had left for Arizona and I was preparing for the second biggest move of my life. I put in a three-week notice at work as I would soon join Steve at Christmas. I was very sad about saying goodbye to the staff and children who had come to mean so much to me. I was not sure I would see them again and our Christmas party was extra special. The last night I saw the kids, I hugged and kissed each one good-bye and told them I loved them. It was strange knowing that they could not understand what I said, but I believed they could feel the warmth I had for them. I was right to anticipate the move west, for a whole new world was about to open up for me.

Chapter Fourteen

FIRST-HAND LOOK

NEW LOVE, new home, new time. I entered 1976 with all these factors in my favor and a very cheerful heart. The arid climate of Arizona greatly helped my physical condition. Within a week the skin sensitivity and itching were much reduced and the stomach pains lessened to the point that I could enjoy a small amount of food and drink. And it was wonderful to be wearing my bathing suit for no other reason than to get a suntan.

This new hope in my heart, that the neuropathy was going away, would help me cope with the latest trauma—impaired vision. What before had been a minor objection in my life was now a major inconvenience. I was not so aware of the large, stringy floaters which had indeed broken up and somewhat dissolved, as Dr. Waring had proposed. But, I did not see better because of this, just differently, and now my eyesight was hazy and blurry. I was still nearsighted and my poor depth perception made seeing things in the distance even more confusing.

I more or less saw things in the general rather than in the specific. I could make out people's faces but could not see wrinkles or the color of their eyes. I could see solid colors of clothing but could not make out patterns or designs. When looking around a room everything looked clean to me, for although I could definitely see furniture in its different colors and shapes, I did not see dust or smoke or even dirt unless it was very obvious. Color contrasts between background and foreground determined a lot of what I could see. For example, I looked right through clear drinking glasses, and it was hard to see a white piece of paper on a white tabletop. On the other hand I could easily see a black piece of clothing on a red couch, even if I wasn't sure what that piece of clothing was. The fewer the objects that were in a room, or on a table, or on a shelf, the easier it was to distinguish between them.

When outside I was a little more apprehensive especially on uneven ground like gravel, or dirt, or grass. I had a real problem with curbs, speed bumps, and holes. I was unable to go up and down steps unless I had a rail or wall to give me balance. I could see trees but not individual leaves.

The more familiar I became with an environment, such as our apartment, the better I was able to get around. The main thing I noticed was that because everything was slightly out of focus, it took my mind longer to interpret what it was I was seeing. Little by little I discovered my limitations and whether to accept them or work around them. The key was patience.

Reading had become extremely difficult. To keep track of phone numbers, addresses, and notes I had to write them with a wide, black magic marker in two-inch high letters. Words written with a ball-point pen, regardless of their size, were simply not dark enough or thick enough for me to easily see.

Mail from family and friends was plentiful, but reading handwriting put a tremendous strain on my eyes. Even letters printed with black, felt-tip pens didn't help much. I loved getting letters and always made an enthusiastic attempt to read them on my own. With my nose pressed against the page, I read only single words or short phrases at a time and in slow staccato. After straining for a couple of paragraphs, Steve would finish reading them to me. I got more out of the letters by listening to his smooth-flowing voice than trying to comprehend the disconnected phrases which I read.

For answering mail, typing was the quickest and easiest. The black type of a typewriter was the only print comfortable for me to read because the letters are small, dark, uniform in size, and spaced evenly apart. I did not take time to proofread, but in concentrating more, I became a better typist.

Whereas in the past I was self-conscious about using a tape recorder, now I readily adapted to this form of communication and began taping cassette letters to my family. This was more personal than letters and saved on phone bills, too. Mother and Grandma were delighted and sent tapes in return.

Steve was a great help to me in many areas. He read or recorded recipes and operating instructions, set the temperature on the oven, and filled all my syringes. On Sundays he entertained me with animated readings of the comics, and I looked forward to his award-winning performances, which provided a lot of laughs.

Cooking went okay as long as I kept things simple, mostly casseroles, meatloafs, and sandwiches—none of these required precise measurements. It was enjoyable to work in the kitchen when I didn't want to eat everything in sight. I even baked brownies and was content to eat just one. At first Steve and I always grocery shopped together, but I was intent on doing something by myself and since I liked this activity more than he did, I decided to solo.

Steve dropped me off at the grocery store one evening and I told him to not pick me up for at least two hours; I wanted to give myself plenty of time. I was carrying a small magnifying glass which Deb had given me. As I made my way down the first aisle, I was eager to accomplish my goal. Stopping at a display of toothbrushes I leaned forward to read the labels, keeping my face within inches of the print in order to focus. I was so absorbed in my task that I jumped slightly when a male voice behind me asked, "What are you doing?"

I whirled around to see a young man about my age, standing there with a curious look on his face. I chuckled and told him I was trying to find a medium toothbrush.

"But what are you doing with that?" he asked, pointing to my magnifying glass.

All of a sudden it dawned on me that because my eyes looked so normal and did not appear to have anything wrong with me, he could not tell I had a vision problem. I explained that I used the glass to read small print and price marks because I could not see well. My words seemed to satisfy him and I turned back to my shopping and was soon again engrossed in my "spy mission."

Two aisles later, the same man—this time accompanied by a young woman—approached me. He asked me if I remembered him and I nodded because I recognized his voice. He introduced the lady as his girlfriend and announced that they were going to help me shop. I smiled at the two, but protested that it was not necessary. But they were so insistent and sincere that I agreed. We proceeded down each aisle, I reading from my large print list, and they running all over filling up my basket. They wanted to know what was wrong with my eyes and when I said I had an eye disease from diabetes, they were very sympathetic. The man kept saying, "Don't worry. We'll take care of you."

We parted at the check-out counter after they were convinced I could pay on my own. I had been touched by their concern and thanked them for their help and time. The two strangers wished me luck and said good-bye.

Upon Dr. Waring's recommendation, I went to see a retina specialist (an ophthalmologist who specializes in diseases of the retina). The specialist told me there was an operation called a vitrectomy in which the fluid in the vitreous is removed and replaced with a clear fluid. In some cases this procedure restores partial or total vision for a person with retinopathy. I was a possible candidate for such an operation although my previous laser surgeries had left some scarring on the retinas, and it could not be helped by a vitrectomy.

I was offered the possibility that the vitrectomy would first be tried on my right eye, which had less vision than my left. Before this could be considered, however, there was a cataract on my right eye which had to be removed so that the doctor could more clearly see the retina and then decide if the vitrectomy would be beneficial.

This news had two effects on Steve and me. For one, it had never been even hinted that I could develop cataracts and mine had apparently grown in the short three months since my last eye exam. On the other hand was the news of the vitrectomy and the miraculous possibility that I might regain perfect vision in at least one of my eyes. Also, the removal of the cataract itself might improve my vision and at worst, it would remain the same. It seemed a small risk for a potentially great reward. I agreed to the plan and Steve gave his full support.

Upon my release from the hospital the ophthalmologist who had been called in to do the surgery, informed me that for the next eight weeks I had to limit most of my physical activity, including no lifting or bending. Luckily, Steve took me for daily walks, but, even so, unbeknownst to me, I began to gain weight for the first time in two years. I was still eating little, but it was obviously more than I needed at the time.

Perhaps I did not notice my gradual weight gain because my thoughts were concentrated on hope of a positive outcome of the surgeries. With half my face covered in an eye patch I sat for hours dreaming of all the things I would do with clear vision. It would be fantastic to read again and, who knows, maybe even drive.

A few weeks after the removal of the eye patch, it was apparent that my vision had not been helped and, in fact, was decreased in the sense that more light now entered my eye and without a lens, I was unable to focus. This did not bother me too much as I relied mostly on my better left eye, and I still had the vitrectomy to look forward to.

Two more months of waiting and hoping, the verdict was delivered in less than five minutes from the retina man. My retina was far too scarred for the risky vitrectomy to do any good. His rejection was so swift and final that I could not say anything. After a stunned pause, I asked if anything at all could be done for my eyes. He said no. As to whether my eyes would stay the same or get worse, he could not say. Both Steve and I were horribly disappointed and we drove home in silence. The ache in my throat kept me from speaking. I was so thankful to have Steve with me — he empathetically squeezed my hand as teardrops ran down my face. It would take a while for this sting to go away.

Thanks to a surprise phone call a couple of weeks later, optimism was again at the forefront of my life. A friend suggested I get in touch with State Service for the Blind, because I may be eligible for money and services. The first thing I needed was certification that I had been legally blind for at least six months. Dr. Waring, in Nebraska, confirmed that the acuity in my good eye (left one) was 20/200 six months previous. It had never occurred to me that I qualified as being "legally blind" — it sounded morbid.

I felt comfortable right away with my new counselor, Anne, who was outgoing and enthusiastic. She said her department's purpose was to provide me with appropriate training and information that would enable me to find employment similar to what I had done before or comparable with my education.

The first step was to get me enrolled in the Skills Center, a state program where I would take courses that would help me adjust to the amount of vision I had. Since the center only accommodated a handful of students at a time, my name was put on a waiting list. Anne also told me I was eligible for monthly checks from Social Security Disability Insurance since I had paid into Social Security for several years.

As eager as I was to start classes, I had something very interesting to fill my time. Anne had initiated me into the Talking Books Program, a nationwide library service for the blind and physically handicapped. This service produces recorded versions by professional readers of books and magazines. These records and cassette tapes are sent back-and-forth through the mail at no cost to the subscribers. Catalogs are also available in recorded and large print editions. Selections include current issues of magazines and books on any topic, past and contemporary.

Anne gave me a special record player which operated at 8 and 16 rpm for the Talking Records. It was mine to keep indefinitely. Anne said the library would also send me headphones and one of the cassette players, called Talking Book Machines.

The joy I felt in reading that first book was indescribable. The book — an exposé of the Patty Hearst story — took ten hours to "read" and I would listen for two to three hours during a sitting, totally absorbed by the voice of the woman who had done the recording. With childlike fascination I was as much enthralled with the story as with the sounds of the words. Her voice was so colorful, it was like listening to a radio play. I especially enjoyed detailed descriptions of scenes.

The more I listened, the more I wanted to saturate myself with words and stories to make up for lost time. It was not only that the Talking Books satisfied my hunger for the printed word, they also helped bring alive a world that was becoming dimmer to me through my own eyes.

The awaited phone call telling me I was to start at the Center came about two months later. I was full of anticipation for what lay ahead and anxious to be busy again. On his way to work Steve drove me to my new "school," which consisted of several trailers and a parking lot. Dave, the mobility instructor, was there to greet me and to introduce me to the staff and other students, an older man and a girl about my age who were both totally blind.

The classes were taught on an individual basis and my schedule included: Home Management; Braille; Arts and Crafts; P.E.: and Mobility and Orientation.

I had chosen Braille as an elective, and I was captivated by the idea of learning to read with my fingertips. The Braille teacher was easygoing and had a unique ability to get concepts across. As with other knowledge, adapting to this "foreign" language took steady work and patience. Forced to learn through my sense of touch, I began to appreciate what it could do for me.

The Home Management class was full of techniques and helpful hints to make cooking and cleaning with impaired vision more safe and enjoyable. One of the first things the teacher taught me was how to open a carton of milk by feeling the top edge and locating the slanted, indented line which indicated that side was the one to open. This simple trick delighted me and to this day, without looking, I can open a carton of milk faster than anyone I know.

I learned that the most important part of cooking is in the planning. Trying to rush just brings frustrations and accidents, to which I could surly testify from my early days in the kitchen. An awareness of sounds and smells is important too, and I saw how vital my nose, ears, and fingers were in cooking, cleaning, and to aid my vision in general.

There are a variety of utensils made especially for blind or visually impaired people. I was given two of them, a Braille kitchen timer and a double pancake turner for turning over meat in a pan without splattering grease. Every few days I would prepare a recipe, practicing the techniques I had been taught.

An important tip for cleaning was to remember to work from side-to-side or from top-to-bottom, such as in wiping a mirror or vacuuming a rug.

Being around the totally blind students gave me an idea of how different it was to learn something with no vision as compared to learning it with partial vision. There was a definite advantage in having gone from perfect vision to partial vision. I could gather enough additional information with my present vision to form a mental picture of what was missing and go on to solve a problem.

On the other extreme, a person blind since birth cannot form mental pictures as a sighted person does, but instead bases his conception on what his other senses tell him. If a handicapped person can't quite grasp an idea, he may feel that his handicap is the sole reason, when actually a lack of vision is only an inconvenience to learning. The mind must understand first and then the body will comply in whatever manner is most conducive. In order to teach the blind or visually impaired, one has to think in those terms.

Mobility and Orientation was my favorite class by far, and gave me confidence in utilizing what vision I had. Much of the credit goes to Dave, the instructor, whom I enjoyed very much. Not only was his sense of humor appealing, but also the demanding, precise way in which he verbally communicated.

The first few days of class Dave and I met in the parking lot to practice "sighted guide" techniques. In my case, I (the follower) walked half-a-step behind and along side of Dave (the guide) while holding on to his bent elbow. The role of the guide was not to give a lot of verbal instructions, but to lead his follower in a safe direction, never pushing the blind person ahead of him. My role was to interpret the physical movements of my guide in dealing with obstacles, changes in elevation, etc. Trust was basic. I had flashbacks of how I had "safely" led George right into a parked car! Steve was a much better guide when leading me into darkened theaters and restaurants.

Dave presented me with a cane on the third day and said it was mine to keep. At first, I thought the idea of me using a cane was ridiculous, because I was nowhere near blind, but I soon learned differently. When I kiddingly referred to it as a "stick," he reprimanded me and said never to refer to it in that way, as all canes were universally alike (black handle, white body, red tip) as a symbol that the person using it has vision problems. The cane was collapsible to a foot in length. The purpose of the cane is as a projection of the arm, hand, and fingers. I quickly adapted to the rhythmical motion of walking with a cane.

When I brought the cane home, Steve immediately wanted to play with it and he kept teasing me by refusing to call the cane anything but a stick!

The weeks that followed were full of challenge and excitement. Dave helped me to understand that the reason a blind or visually impaired person can learn to mobilize so well is because he learns to develop and use concentration and memory — two essential tools. People with good vision often rely only on their sight and don't make use of these other abilities. Of course, that is one of the advantages of vision itself. But for a sight-impaired person, forgetting to feel for steps in a certain area, for example, could result in an accident.

The other important aspect of travel, with or without a cane, is the use of landmarks, which are anything a person uses to help remind him where he is. There was one fast rule — landmarks must be stable. For instance, buildings are good, as are signs, fences, and trees, because they are not likely to be moved. Dave said never to use parked cars, fenced in or chained animals, or things that could change location at any time.

Sounds, too, can be landmarks: churchbells; loud-speakers; music coming from a record store; or elevator doors opening and closing. My sense of smell told me if I was near a shoe repair shop, a drug store, or a bakery. Shadows not only help determine time of day of year, but provide contrasts to aid in depth perception. My power of observation increased and it was fun looking for and using familiar environmental clues.

Dave drove me to quiet neighborhoods, city office buildings, and shopping malls where I could practice letting my cane "see" for me. Soon I became comfortable going up-and-down curbs, dealing with obstructions, and locating specific places or buildings on my own. Dave emphasized that I not be shy about asking others for directions, requesting that they be exact — two blocks north and one block west, rather than a few blocks over there.

The day came when Dave told me I was ready to cross the busiest intersection in Phoenix all by myself. He stood observing, a few feet away, but did nothing to help me. I was nervous, for sure, but I knew I could do it because I had learned "defensive walking."

Rather than looking at the traffic lights, which I could not see anyway, I watched the sequence of the flow of cars. I first paid attention to whoever might be making a turn in front of me. Then as the general flow of traffic moved into the intersection going the same way I was, I stepped from the curb and quickly made my way across, tapping my cane from side-to-side as I walked. When I neared the opposite side I made contact with my cane at the curb so I would know where to step up. It went smooth as silk and I tingled with excitement.

Learning to ride a bus was next on my mobility agenda. It incorporated most of the techniques I had learned and would allow me to get around the many miles of Phoenix. First I trained on an empty bus — getting on and off and finding a seat. Next, Dave familiarized me with the main bus terminal downtown. Then he gave me the number of the bus I was to catch. It would take me to the bus stop near my home, where Dave would be waiting.

As each bus pulled up, I inquired what number it was. There was a mob of people and I got flustered and missed my bus all together. Embarrassed, I stepped back to wait the half hour for the next bus. I knew Dave would never let me hear the end of it. Suddenly I heard a voice say, "Wanna ride home?" I turned to see Dave grinning. He had witnessed the entire event from across the street.

The next day, after boarding the right bus, Dave was waiting at the other end to congratulate me. He said with this particular achievement I had successfully passed his class, and I was now on my own to practice and put what I had learned to good use.

My two months of schooling was over. The teachers and the classes had given me more than just some useful techniques. They had given me a sense of freedom and I was ready to fly!

Chapter Fifteen

IN BETWEEN

LEARNING TO GET around with my cane was like being reborn. As when I had learned to drive a car, a whole world was brought within my reach. I felt so independent, which is the most important way a handicapped person can feel.

I began going to the grocery store by myself and even to doctor's appointments and shopping centers across town. Steve was very proud of me. I was happy to be taking some of the burden of transporting me off of him, even though he gladly took me wherever I wanted to go.

Physically, I was doing so well that even my appetite returned to normal — normal for me that is. Steve would sometimes kid me about how much I ate but never said anything derogatory. I think he was relieved to see me eating again after so many months of distaste for food.

With others, the fact that I ate a lot got little attention. People were far more attracted to my cane and my visual difficulties. My identification as a diabetic shifted to my new role — that of being visually impaired.

My advantage, of course, was that I was not totally blind, and the more I mobilized, the more I got used to getting around with the vision I did have. It was an unusual position to be in. People would place me in either of two categories — perfectly sighted or blind. Actually, I fell somewhere in between and this is what others did not seem to comprehend.

One reason for this dual label was that when others looked at me, they saw normal eyes. They could not tell that the view I had was like looking at a very snowy picture on T.V. with millions of minute black dots dispersed throughout my field of vision. Also, when I was talking to someone I forced myself to look straight in his eyes, which meant that I could not see them. The only way I could see the eyes was to look slightly off center at the nose or mouth. This was because my peripheral (side) vision was so much sharper than my center vision.

Dave had been the one who suggested I at least give the impression I was looking at someone's eyes to make them more comfortable looking at me, and I found this to be true.

If I was indoors with my cane folded up and my sunglasses off, people would hesitate to help me if I asked for directions or help in reading a sign. Presumably, this was because I looked as if I could see. On the other hand, when I was outside and had my cane in front of me and sunglasses on, strangers treated me as blind since I really looked the part.

Occasionally, I took advantage of people when they assumed I could not see anything. If someone allowed me to go first in line or take the only empty seat on a bus, I would not protest. The majority of people were sincere and wanted to help.

Once I was at a stoplight watching for the sequence of lights to run through so I could start across the moment the light turned green. All of a sudden, a voice from the other side of the street yelled, "You can go now!"

On the other hand, since I had to be so aware of everything, I also was in the position to notice how unaware other people were, especially motorists. Many a time it was my vision—not my cane—that saved me from smacking into a car that was jutting over the line of an intersection.

The cane was now in the other hand, so to speak, and I saw people doing to me what I had done to handicapped people in the past. An individual coming toward me down the street would wait until 15 or so feet in front of me and then make an abrupt wide arc to avoid me. Sometimes I would smile broadly and say, "Hi!", knowing he thought I couldn't see, but just to note his reaction. At the same time though, I empathized with his feelings of discomfort.

The bus drivers of Phoenix were friendly to me and helpful in giving directions and calling out the names of major streets as we approached them. It was the hours of waiting on bus stops and the transferring that got to me once in a while. I very much appreciated the fact that I was entitled to a bus pass allowing me to ride anytime and anywhere for free.

The passengers on a bus were another story. According to whether or not they saw my cane and sunglasses, they would either ignore me and act self-conscious if I sat by them, or they would treat me normally and carry on a conversation.

Each day that I went out with my cane was an adventure if only because I did not know what unexpected thing would happen next. The awkward times when I felt unsure of myself, gratefully, were offset with humorous situations. My favorite recollection was the time I met my friend Mel at the courthouse to attend the public hearings of a murder trial. As soon as we were inside, I folded up my cane and slipped it into Mel's large purse. We happened to be sitting directly behind the defendant.

During the first recess, Mel and I were dumbfounded when the district attorney escorted us out of the courtroom and into a private office. There a female police officer took us inside a closet-sized room and searched our purses. As Mel demanded to know what was going on, I broke out in nervous goose bumps. The officer explained in a stern voice that someone had seen us put a large metal object into a purse.

Mel looked confused, but I chuckled, remembering my cane. I told the officer I was visually impaired and carried a cane. She was not as amused as we were at the mishap and told us we were barred from the courtroom, because our presence made the jury uneasy. I couldn't believe what had happened, and I didn't even mind the eviction since it gave me a great story to relate to family and friends.

Another girl I became friends with was a student from the Skills Center, Carol. After discovering that we only lived a mile apart, we took turns walking to each other's homes or meeting at a Sambo's for coffee and a chat. We learned from one another and, together, got into some hilarious circumstances. Like the time we were on a bus, missed our stop because we were talking, and ended up in a part of town neither of us knew. When we realized what had happened, the concerned bus driver — dragging Carol and me behind him — crossed right in the middle of a very busy street to reach the bus stop we needed. All that had been necessary were some simple, verbal directions. As the poor driver dashed back to his waiting bus, Carol and I burst out laughing.

At Carol's encouragement, I joined her bowling league for the blind and visually impaired. I had thought it would be embarrassing to be amidst an entire group of blind people sharing an activity, but my prejudgment could not have been more wrong. As it turned out, I had great fun with this group and it was nice not having to explain when I could not see something — it was just understood. In the near future, my involvement with the league would bring even bigger payoffs.

At other times I resented being placed automatically in the world of the blind. One morning, an instructor from the Skills Center showed up at our apartment to mark our stove with Braille symbols that would indicate various temperature settings. The living room, although not dirty, needed straightening up. The teacher made no comment on the disarray and proceeded to do what she had come for.

Later my counselor, Anne, told me that the teacher had remarked to her that my living room was messy and perhaps I needed more training in housecleaning. Having been in the homes of other blind people, I knew at once why the teacher reacted as she did. Most of them keep their homes meticulously neat out of practicality and necessity, and naturally do not have books, papers, and such lying around. They need to be able to move about freely and find things out of habit, whereas sighted people can manage to find things no matter how disorganized they are. Cleaning up, or not, is a matter of individual preference if you can see.

Here I was, not fitting the mold of what most blind people do. Had I known in advance she was coming, I would have quickly picked up, leaving her with exactly the opposite impression — that I was quite capable of keeping a neat house, which I was. It annoyed me that my low vision had been blamed for what was just a personality trait.

The truth was that I made a real attempt to continue the same amount of cleaning that I had done with perfect vision. I never wanted an easy excuse not to do things. This desire to remain "normal" led to frustrating as well as comical scenarios.

Once I nearly burned out the motor of a vacuum because I had sucked up some socks I had not seen lying on the carpet. After that, I always went around on all fours checking for objects before I turned on the vacuum.

My girlfriend, Vicki, was visiting from Nebraska when another episode with the vacuum occurred. She walked into the bedroom where I was busily pushing a vacuum back-and-forth and she asked where all the dust was coming from. Not knowing what she was talking about, I continued what I was doing.

Suddenly Vicki burst out laughing and at the same time grabbed the machine from me and shut it off. I questioned what she was doing, but she was laughing so hard she couldn't speak. Finally, between chuckles, she got out that the door to the dust trap had opened up and each time I moved the vacuum in any direction, I sent dirt and dust flying. She said I had looked so innocent, working away in a cloud of dust that I was oblivious to!

Every month or so I noticed a slight decrease in my vision. The changes may have been insignificant to a person with better vision, but to me, each change was apparent and disheartening and adjusting to them was an ongoing process. I wondered if there was anyone else who saw the world the way I did, and I was becoming more empathetic with people who had handicaps of any kind.

My vision changes were also being followed by psychological turmoil and analysis on my part. There was such a dichotomy of feelings within me. On the one hand, there were the interesting things I was learning, the humorous incidents, the awareness of my ability to cope with new situations, and my associations with other handicapped people. On the other hand, I sensed a feeling of resentment at what was happening to me.

Although I cannot speak about other senses, losing part of my vision seemed to have a grief process all its own. I had read a book about the stages people go through in accepting their own inevitable death or the death of a loved one. I knew I was experiencing similar stages. My feelings were not clear cut and moved back-and-forth among self-pity, resistance, and acceptance.

Because I believed that everyone around me could see perfectly, I assumed it was their duty to explain to me whatever I could not see. In the time I had spent with Dave, he had been so thorough in describing objects and scenes to me that I became that much more aware of what I was missing. I expected others to be equally as exact in their descriptions. Luckily, Steve picked up where Dave left off and was acutely sensitive to my desire to have the pieces of my visual pictures completed. Having been a newspaper reporter for so many years, he had trained himself to be observant and he became superb at painting pictures for my mind to absorb. I relied heavily on him.

The inaccuracies of other people were understandable since they were not accustomed to defining what they saw with such clarity. Nevertheless, I found myself getting impatient with them and sometimes I even thought people were deliberately keeping visual information from me. If others talked about something I could not see, I constantly asked questions, which I'm sure was annoying. I often felt left out and, consequently, less of a person.

For example, I did not like looking at photographs because I could not see details and therefore became bored. I was jealous of what others could see beyond what I did.

Also, I was tense while watching television with others as they could catch actions or details that I often missed. If someone with me laughed or the T.V. audience laughed, and I did not know why, I practically demanded to know what was so funny. I preferred to view with those who gave me a running commentary of what was happening or just being by myself and not knowing what or if I had missed anything.

When I was with Carol, I thought I could see the moon by comparison. At these times I had the role of describing and explaining to her. But she did not seem to feel as left out as I did in similar situations. She had never known what it was she was not seeing, while I was still getting used to being visually teased and wanting more.

Probably the most difficult, yet vital area of change was learning to communicate with people in a new way. Before this, I had not realized how much of our communication and interaction is done with our eyes and our vision. I was no longer able to detect subtle eye and facial expressions and often felt like a radio receiver which is not picking up any signals or is picking up weak ones.

Out of necessity, I gradually began to rely on information from my other senses, as I did when mobilizing. I observed gross motor movements, refined my hearing to intense listening, often used my intuition, and became more attentive to the nonverbal messages of body language.

Many times I misinterpreted the signals or was slow in reading them. It drove me crazy when quiet people would nod or shake their heads instead of speaking, as I relied so heavily on tone, inflection, and other voice qualities. Talkative and/or demonstrative persons gave me a lot to work with and attracted my attention.

It was an odd feeling to know that others could see my face better than I could see it. Even when looking into a mirror, I saw only my blurred image.

More enjoyable than ever now was talking on the phone because no vision was necessary and I was equal to the person on the other end. I may even have had a slight advantage in that I not only listened more closely to what a person said, but also how he said it.

It was not unusual for friends and relatives to ask: is it true that losing one sense makes the other senses stronger? The answer is no — at least not automatically. Any person has the potential to develop and make use of any of his senses at any time. But because vision supplies so much information and is the most consciously used sense, people rely the most on it. A visually impaired or blind person sort of switches gears, using data from other sources which was always available but seldom used. It is all a matter of necessary adaptation.

Relating nonvisually to people has its risks; I have put my foot in my mouth on many occasions when I did not fully realize the circumstances of a situation and did not show patience in finding them out. It was embarrassing to have made a comment about someone thinking he was not there or not within earshot, and then finding out he was. If someone was with me at the time and my mistake proved to be humorous, I just laughed at myself. But if I caused awkwardness for someone else, I was angry and ashamed and my limitations made me feel handicapped.

Chapter Sixteen

FAMILY TIES AND KNOTS

THE FIRST member of my family to see me after my graduation from the Skills Center was Lisa. She and a girlfriend drove up one weekend from Albuquerque, and I was anxious to show off what I had learned. Lisa had been to visit before my classes so I knew she would be seeing a whole new me.

While I was still living at home, I had never been close to Lisa, partly because of the six years difference in our ages. But mostly because while the three of us were growing up, Deb and I were constantly together and did not have much time for her. Now Lisa was 18 and out on her own, and her visits drew us together as good friends. She had been a little girl when I left for college, but now she seemed more like a peer and I enjoyed getting to know her. She was sincerely interested in my eye problems and I was impressed with her mature attitude. She never pitied me, but accepted me and attempted to understand what I was dealing with. To this day we share a special closeness.

Predictably, she was very enthusiastic about the skills I had acquired. She and her friend listened to all the details and were intrigued by my Abacus, Braille workbook, and Braille watch. Like Steve, they both had a wonderfully humorous reaction to the whole thing and they laughed at the many anecdotes about my vision. Lisa was so amazed that I could get around the city on my own and her expressions of praise and confidence made me feel so good about myself.

With Deb I was a little more anxious to show her all I had learned and how good I could get around. I knew that she too, like the rest of my family, felt bad about my vision loss and would be glad to see how independent I had become.

Since I had moved to Arizona we wrote letters and talked frequently on the phone. This had been the first time in our lives that we had been separated for more than a month and I was feeling close to her and believed our relationship to be intimate once again. Whenever she was depressed or troubled, she would call to ask for my advice or just to share her feelings. Absence had seemed to make her heart grow fonder, and I anticipated a reunion between us.

I had been gone a year when I flew back to Nebraska to attend the wedding of my college roommate, Patrice, and to visit Deb. Deb arrived in Omaha with a group of friends to pick me up. She acted so casual and indifferent that I was a bit stunned. It was not the meeting I had expected, but I tried to act natural and friendly. I showed the girls my cane and made a joke, trying to set a light tone. Deb did not inquire about the cane or its use, so I said nothing, sensing that perhaps she felt awkward and did not know how to react to me. Although I had talked to her extensively about the cane on the phone, maybe the actual sight of it was too much in that it brought to reality the meaning of my partial loss of sight. I thought it best to take it easy and let her initiate the general topic.

Over the next few days of my visit I found that my old friends were very interested in all I had learned at the school. At first I was somewhat inhibited about using my cane in front of them because I thought they would compare me to the way I was before. But as soon as they realized that I took it all with a sense of humor, they followed suit. Several remarked that I was getting around so much better than the last time they had seen me and wanted to know if I was seeing better. I explained that my eyes had not improved but that I was more effectively using what vision I had. This fact amazed them.

Even though I was staying at Deb's apartment, I saw little of her. Her work and other activities kept her busy, but I figured that before I left, we would engage in a heart-to-heart sisterly talk and share what was going on in our lives. However, we never did have the hoped for talk and anytime we did spend together was uneasy and superficial. It became more apparent as time passed that she wished to avoid any discussion relating to vision.

Whenever we went somewhere together, she was overly protective about my mobility, especially when we were going up-and-down steps or curbs. She would not wait to see that with a little extra time, I could get around fine. She had always been quick in her actions and movements and my need for a little patience made her nervous. She was not alone in her behavior — I noticed that many people treat handicapped individuals like this, assuming it is safer and faster to do things themselves rather than to wait and see how the handicapped person will deal with the situation. They forget that we have to learn to do things with as little help as possible.

Deb, instead of slowing down, would ask me every few minutes if I was all right, or she would apologize when I stumbled the least little bit. My handicap either scared her or made her feel uncomfortable and she took the role of protector. I should have told her that even seeing eye dogs work with blind people and do not just take over for them. I excused her attitude because I thought that past exposures to my diabetic problems probably influenced her feelings that I could not take care of myself.

Inside her apartment, the situation was no better. It was a new place to me and I did not know where things were kept. Before asking her, though, I would try to think logically where she might keep a certain item. When I did ask, her answers were broad and generalized such as, "It's in the hall cabinet." Her hall cabinet was loaded with stuff and I had to be careful when going through it. If I asked her to be more specific, she would jump up and get the item herself. Each time I was shown the location of something, I made a mental note of it. But inevitably other questions came up.

Deb was exasperated and finally said to me, "All these months you've been telling me how good you can get around your apartment and how good you are seeing, but you seem so helpless around me."

Her words stung, but I tried to remain calm as I explained that I could get around my apartment as fast as anyone because I always put things in the same place and knew exactly where they were. Naturally, in an unfamiliar place, I had to learn the arrangement of things and that took time. She may have heard my words, but not their implication, for she continued to act annoyed.

Unfortunately, my mobility was not the only sore spot between us. It had been so long since anyone hassled me about my eating habits that when Deb began nagging me about what I ate and not taking care of myself, I was quite taken aback. After all the time that had gone by and our compatible long-distance relationship, she was returning to her "mother" role and it was like high school and college all over again. I tried brushing off her comments, not believing she would keep them up as a barrier between us. But, I was mistaken and her constant remarks about food led to a bitter argument one day in front of a friend. I was hurt and humiliated.

Later, in private, I could no longer hold back, and I told Deb that we were grown up now and could not continue to act as we had in the past. I was responsible for my own actions and did not question what she did, and I saw no reason why we couldn't treat each other like adults. I begged her to please be open and tell me what was going on.

It was no use trying to talk to her — she became defensive and started yelling at me. She stood up and began rearranging things on the coffee table and picking up the living room in an obvious attempt to put off a discussion. Nothing was being settled and I finally gave up in despair.

After that confrontation, I could not wait to leave town. Deb informed me she would not be able to drive me to the airport and I would have to make other plans. When the time came we did not even hug good-bye, and the air was thick with uneasiness and bitterness. We bid farewell as if we hardly knew one another.

During the flight back I was numb and did not even cry, but there was an empty, sick feeling in my stomach. When Steve picked me up, he knew right away that something was wrong for I was not the cheerful, happy person who had left him. He listened while I briefly told him about the trip and the way Deb had acted, admitting that I no longer felt close to her and doubted my love for her. Worst of all, it did not bother me that I felt this way. I was hurt too deeply to feel pain.

For the next many months, I was not sad that neither Deb nor I wrote or called. Years later she would confide in me that this had been a particularly troubled period in her life with male relationships and work problems. But at the time, her attitude was something I could only surmise. I contemplated about what had happened and was even able to view our estrangement as an objective onlooker. She had not handled my diabetes too well and my vision problems just complicated matters. Maybe she felt guilty because I had health problems and she did not, or maybe my physical handicap embarrassed her. There were plenty of people who accepted me as I was and I had to realize that she was not one of them.

Four months later, when we finally talked on the phone, it was like nothing had happened. She called me and we got along beautifully. She was friendly and chatty, inquiring about how Steve and I were doing. I was both pleased and puzzled by this return to our former rapport. Then it came to me that as long as we were apart, we could have a good relationship. By writing letters or talking on the phone, she could not see me or what I was doing. We were equals and she did not have to deal with my diabetes or vision. Whether or not she was aware of this, I could accept it.

In the future, whenever I was with her, such as at Christmas, I had to take what came and not expect too much from her. An unexpected turn of events enhanced our closeness. She got a new job as a counselor in an alcoholic treatment program and became very involved. She confessed to me that she was beginning to understand our strained relationship a little better. She said authorities in her field often compared alcoholism to diabetes in areas such as the outreaching effects on the family, friends, and peers, the tremendous guilt experienced by the person, and the consequences on other parts of the person's life when the disease is not controlled. Deb said she had never looked at diabetes as causing emotional or psychological problems.

Pleased with her insight, I agreed, and I admitted that I often thought it would be easier to be alcoholic because then it would just be a matter of stopping drinking whereas, with diabetes, I could not stop eating. It was an ongoing situation I had to deal with. This was the first time, I believe, that Deb was looking objectively at the diabetes and how it influenced our family relationships: she and me, and me and the rest of the family.

Not long after my visit with Deb in Nebraska, I decided to fly home and see the remainder of my family in New Mexico. Despite what had transpired between Deb and me, I was eager to show the others what I had learned. Mother, of course, was delighted to see me and was so impressed that I could get around. She had a loving, accepting attitude as well as a sense of humor about my problems and my willingness to adapt. She trusted me completely to do anything, or go wherever I wanted with my cane, and she praised me often.

I was so used to Mother's cheery voice on the telephone and her upbeat letters, that I sometimes forgot about her arthritis, which had become progressively worse over the past ten years. Her fingers were permanently bent, she could not kneel or bend very much at the knee, and she was unable to reach for anything higher than shoulder level. The pain in all her joints was severe and it was unending, but I never heard her complain.

After enjoying Mother's company for a few days, I took a bus down south to visit Grandma in Truth or Consequences. Mother would follow in the car on the weekend to pick me up. I had not seen Grandma in over a year since moving to Phoenix, and my vision had changed quite a bit. She had heard all about my surgeries and my classes, and I think she must have pictured in her mind that things were worse than they really were. Like Deb, Grandma did not want to see what I could do. She did not want me to do anything around the house, either, for fear I would not be able to do what I attempted or that I would hurt myself. Many people were like Grandma, assuming that no vision, or little vision, automatically means accidents and upsets.

Here I was, fresh out of school and feeling so confident, and she saw me only as a blind and helpless person. We had some mild arguments over this and I knew she was afraid for me out of ignorance. But also, I knew that if she gave me a chance, I could prove my capabilities.

I explained to Grandma that I could do practically anything if I was just careful and methodical. She finally gave in out of exasperation and not because she was convinced. To make up for lost time, I ironed a basket of clothes, cleaned her entire house, and did some cooking. It did the trick. She praised me up-and-down and kept saying she didn't know how I did it.

One day, after Mother had arrived, I told Grandma that I planned to walk to the Circle K that was six blocks from her home and added that I would not have to cross any busy streets. "Of course not!" she objected. Luckily, Mother came to my defense and said I could do it and for Grandma to let me go. So, I set off, cane in hand, with Grandma watching me out the living room window. I returned a short while later bearing my purchase to prove that I had been successful. Again, Grandma was amazed, and slowly but surely, she began to trust me and all that I could do.

At times she even showed her sense of humor about my vision loss. I remember she owned a clear glass ashtray. After a meal, we'd each have a cigarette. Once, I laid my cigarette directly on the table, thinking it was the ashtray. Grandma thought the mistake was so funny and we both started laughing. She said nothing about the burn mark left on her beautiful dining room table. She continues to acknowledge how well I use my vision and even says I see better than she does, which I know is not true, but it makes me feel pretty good anyway.

Another surprising change in Grandma came to my attention—she no longer said anything about what I ate. After Deb's reaction, I had expected a similar one from Grandma. Ironically, though, she had been recently diagnosed as having high blood sugars, and she had immediately put herself on a diet. She eventually lost over 20 pounds which she has not regained, and her blood sugars have returned to normal. Years later, I would read that it is not uncommon for overweight people who have slimmed down to no longer have the symptoms of diabetes. Because of this, perhaps she now emphasized and/or figured I had enough to cope with in my life without more nagging.

Mealtimes with Grandma were now very pleasant, and I know she was relieved to have someone helping with the cooking. I no longer resented the little bowls of vegetables which she still placed around my plate, because it was a whole new atmosphere.

Something else happened on this trip which had a special meaning for my life. At Grandma's house, she had her own bedroom, and guests always slept in the front bedroom on twin beds. Mother and I were sharing this room, and one night as we lay in our beds, we talked of things we had never before discussed. I asked her if, because of the pain she suffered with for so many years, she ever doubted her belief in God? She said yes. Then we talked a long time about our diseases and how they were different, and yet alike, how they affected our lives, and how they made us question things.

I told Mother that what I went through seemed so easy compared to what she went through, and she told me just the opposite. We were appreciating each other in a new, meaningful way because we shared what the rest of the family had not known and probably never would. We were comrades in a often unpredictable, frustrating world and found security in knowing there was someone who had true empathy. I felt so close to her from then on.

That night I silently cried myself to sleep, thinking of how much I loved Mother and how much I hated the constant pain she was in. I wanted so much to be able to provide her with answers and to relieve her suffering. Little did either of us know how soon our lives would change and how much closer our paths would come together.

Back home in Phoenix, I heard on a radio talk show about an extension class being offered through Arizona State University. The professor of the class had been so interesting on the talk show, that I was eager to sign up. The class was called Suicide, Death, and Dying, and for some reason sounded very intriguing to me. I enrolled and found that taking the class proved to be a significant turning point in my life, for I was exposed to ideas and conditions I had never thought of before. Just meeting the members of my class was an experience in itself. One was a funeral director, one was a nurse who worked with terminally ill children, and several others were widows or widowers of suicide or natural death victims.

Part of our assignment was to read as many books as possible from a special reading list prepared by the professor. What books were not on Talking Books, I was able to have put on cassettes by Recording for the Blind, a nationwide organization in which volunteers record textbooks for visually impaired or blind students.

The books covered suicide, death, and dying, from a variety of perspectives — physical, mental, philosophical, and spiritual. It was the reading of books that sparked something inside of me, and long after the class ended, I continued to read countless books on those and similar topics. I began to look at diabetes and vision problems from a psychological/philosophical angle for the first time, and I wondered why I had these particular conditions. Why me? It was not that I ever thought I did not deserve the problems, but I was daring to think a lot about them.

All of this remained in the back of my mind as I began to explore unorthodox forms of healing, relaxation techniques, mind control, and Yoga. For awhile, I took biofeedback sessions and enjoyed the mental exercise of visualization. I felt my awareness expanding like it never had before, and I derived a certain comfort for coping with my problems. It was not a punishment or sin type of awareness, but more like my problems had brought me to a new crossroads in my life. I realized with amazement that my loss of vision had led me to Talking Books, which led me to hours of reading, time I may never have taken had my vision remained perfect.

While my outlook had dimmed, my "inlook" had brightened. My experiences were those not everyone would have, and I felt special in my own way.

Coincidence or not, about this time Mother sent me tapes to listen to that were relevant to the areas I had been studying, even though I had not told her of my new interest. I was thrilled to know that she, too, was open-minded and I would be able to communicate with her about the ideas I was reading and contemplating. In the months that followed, we shared everything we thought would appeal to the other. We were being drawn away from the closed-in, limiting, nonsensical atmosphere of living with chronic diseases. It was as if a common thread had been discovered and was bringing us closer together in a beautiful way.

Chapter Seventeen

A MIRACLE

WITH MY mobility and skills training behind me, it was time to forge ahead with the purpose of the training, to find employment. I so looked forward to work, to feeling useful and productive again, and to prove that I could do something valuable to earn money. I knew that working would add a new, fulfilling dimension to my living as a visually impaired person. But, I did not know that it would be my life outside of work which would channel the opening of a truly exciting and promising world for me.

Finding me work was now the job of my counselor, Anne. Not only did the work have to be in the area of my education and previous experience, it also had to be in an area where my vision was not a deterrent. We talked it over and agreed that if I could work part-time at some sort of teaching job, I would be able to determine how much more I could handle. Anne phoned one day with news of a part-time position opening up at a preschool for deaf/blind children.

Steve and I went to check out the school, since I did have a say in whether or not I accepted the job. The class I was to be in had kids with mental and physical handicaps in addition to vision and hearing losses. I felt well qualified to work with them, so arrangements were made for me to start two months later at the beginning of the spring semester, 1977.

Boy, was I feeling fantastic as I rode a bus to the first job I'd had in one-and-a-half years. I was ready to accomplish great things. One thing that had attracted me to the school was that two of the workers also had vision problems — one girl blind since birth, and another girl visually impaired for many years. Knowing the longevity of their conditions, I liked to observe and learn from how smoothly they got around.

Like the children Steve and I had worked with in Nebraska, these kids, too, required one-to-one teaching and I enjoyed them very much.

122

They ranged in ages from six to 12 and had varying degrees of vision and hearing loss. Throughout each day I would pay close attention to the teacher's methods, taking mental notes for possible use in the future. Although the teacher, who was my age, was excellent at planning activities and setting program goals for the students, she had one very annoying personality flaw. Her way of dealing with blindness and visual impairment was to make crude remarks and jokes. I got the impression she was insecure and probably believed that she was displaying a good sense of humor. But with her you got the feeling she was not laughing with you but at you.

She'd call her aide, who was blind, "Blinko" and other names, and if the aide or I dropped something on the floor, the teacher would yell, "Get down on the floor and feel for it!" I had never been ridiculed before and her treatment of us was quite unnerving. The only reason I could put up with this person was because I liked the work, and because of John, another aide, who had a genuine humorous attitude and a good-natured personality.

My time away from work was integrated with Talking Books, sun-tanning, and recreational pastimes. And I was still bowling with the league, never dreaming that the most incredible moment of my life was about to take place in a bowling alley.

Carol and I were substituting one Saturday for two absentee bowlers on another team. One of our teammates was a middle-aged, visually impaired woman, who was wearing glasses and appeared to be seeing quite well. We were talking about our eye problems and she said that for a long time she had not seen very well. Then she found a doctor who prescribed the glasses she now wore, and they made all the difference in the world. She could even read very small print. I was happy for her discovery. She kept urging me to try on her glasses, and I kept refusing because I often tried on others' glasses and none of them made any difference in my eyesight.

Finally, I decided to put them on, more out of curiosity than hope. As I slipped them on I almost jumped back in surprise—it was a miracle! All around me bright colors seemed to jump out of nowhere. I cried out with joy, "I can see! Carol, I can see and everything is so bright!"

It was like looking through a child's kaleidoscope in which the colors and shapes seem to move around and do not make complete pictures, but rather designs. As I surveyed the room, I caught glimpses of people's faces and letters on signs. This distortion did not bother me, nor the fact that my left eye was in focus and my right eye was blurry—it was all magnificent! I tried to absorb everything at once and never wanted to take those glasses off.

I had lost interest in bowling for the day. The discovery was so wonderful, it had to be true. Each time the woman completed her turn, I would ask to try on the glasses again to prove I wasn't dreaming. She and Carol were delighted and told me I should try to get a pair of the glasses. I had already decided that, the instant I tried them on.

When my ride dropped me off at our apartment, I raced upstairs and flew into the living room and tried to blurt out the entire story to Steve in one breath. Steve remained calm, but I knew he was thrilled for me. He said we would immediately find a way to get a pair of the glasses.

So began the search. I figured the first step was to contact the doctor who had removed my cataract a year earlier. He listened quietly and then had me sit in front of a machine which had interchanges of various strengths of lenses. I insisted again that with my friend's glasses, colors were vivid and I was able to read large letters on signs.

When the doctor next spoke, I felt like a child being reprimanded by an all-knowing adult. He shook his head from side-to-side and said, "Denise, you just think you see better with those glasses, but you don't." I looked at him in astonishment. His comment insinuated that I had stretched the truth because I so desperately wanted to believe it. I made no reply, not wanting to dignify his words with a response.

Steve and I left in disgust and I thought how wonderful Steve was. He had not seen the glasses either, but he had believed and trusted that what I said was true. Despite the doctor's indifference to helping me, Steve and I were more determined than ever to succeed.

Next, I phoned the woman who owned the glasses hoping she would offer to loan me them to show my doctor, but instead she gave me the name of her eye doctor and said I could use her name for reference. Two more weeks elapsed before I could meet with her doctor. He was very hesitant about "discussing another patient's case." I couldn't believe all this secrecy over a prescription for glasses. After much pleading on mine and Steve's part to at least write down the type of glasses they were, he finally scribbled a note and handed it to me. When Steve and I were outside, he read the note, which simply said "cataract lenses." We had no idea what they were but it sounded logical since I had had a cataract operation.

Even with the note, it was like pulling teeth to get my doctor to write a prescription. He insisted that getting the glasses would be a waste of time and money—they would do nothing for me. I told him I did not care about the time or money and that I had to find out for myself. He reluctantly wrote what I wanted, but with no word of hope or good luck.

Anne was elated about the news and directed me to the Low Vision Clinic. No appointment was necessary and Steve and I rushed over. A technician brought out several pairs of glasses and told me to try one of them on. He placed a printed card in front of me to test my visual acuity for reading. I was to move the card toward and away from my face. It was all a blur. The man put a second pair on me and moved the card closer to my face. Back-and-forth . . . blurry . . . blurry. I wanted to see more than anything. All of a sudden a word on the card became clear and I exclaimed out loud that I could see it. This was great! I had hoped to see around a room, but now I was doubly blessed. I read an entire sentence in slow, jerky phrases, but it was music to my ears and eyes. Glancing up, I saw the beautiful, distorted colors and shapes. To think I had been missing all these magnificent sights for more than a year — I was so thankful for the chance to see them again.

The technician suggested I get bifocals, which would allow me the most vision for walking and reading. I picked out frames and within a week I was wearing my very own magic glasses. I quickly discovered that it was like having hand held magnifying glasses in front of my eyes — unless I stood still, it was hard to focus, and walking or riding made me nauseous. Also the thickness of the lenses allowed in so much sunlight that it hurt my eyes, and the high magnification factor made objects appear larger than normal and closer to my body. Having grown used to the way I saw without glasses, I was now clumsy again at mobilizing. My "miracle" would certainly take some getting used to, but I was willing to make the adjustment.

I was anxious to wear the glasses to work and knew they would help me do a better job. The first day I had them on I was a little self-conscious, because the thick glass made my eyes appear noticeably larger. As soon as the teacher saw me in them, she called me "four eyes" and continued to refer to them as "pop bottles." Had she suspended her comments after that first day I probably would have forgotten them, but she kept up the teasing. I was painfully embarrassed and could not take her words with a sense of humor, as I likely would have if John had made them.

No one else, including strangers, made fun of me or called me names, and, in fact, most people I knew who saw me in them praised the glasses and the better vision they provided me. So, why was I so affected by the teacher's attitude? I started to feel odd and almost freaky. When I confided to Steve about my insecurities, he rebuked me, saying that I must think very little of myself if how I looked to others was more important than seeing better. My eyes moistened with tears, because he had acknowledged that the problem came from within me.

But, whether it was vanity or not, I did care how I looked and if people stared at me. I had allowed one person's reaction blow my self-image out of proportion. At school, I refrained from wearing the glasses, except to pick up the crumbs off the floor at lunchtime. Gradually, I wore them less for general seeing and walking outside. Although I missed the bright colors and detail, I did walk more smoothly without the glasses, since my depth perception would be normal.

By no means had I stopped enjoying the glasses. Inside our apartment I wore them for watching television, filling up my insulin syringes, and reading and writing. I think reading was the most fun; I wanted to go to a library and not leave until I had read every book in the place.

After several weeks of eagerly using my expanded vision, there was a marked increase of blurriness in my eyes. My first instinct was to ignore it, knowing that a diabetic's eyes can blur randomly from changes in blood sugar. But the condition persisted and I thought it was time to see the retina specialist again. My doctor was out of the country for two months, so I met with his partner. After waiting several hours, I finally saw the doctor. He was in a terrible hurry and I barely had time to capsulize my eye condition and why my ophthalmologist had wanted me to come in. He made no reply and quickly looked into my eyes with some instruments. Then he mumbled something about my eyes being "end out," a term I had never heard. I asked about its meaning and he started yelling at me and saying that my eyes were not changing, would never change again, and I had to accept them as they were.

Trying to retain my composure I told him that I was not aware that the disease could just end, as no other doctor had mentioned it. He snarled back, "You're just going to have to stop being an ocular cripple!"

His outburst scared and upset me for I had no idea what he was referring to. I was unable to speak and stared at him in disbelief. Adding insult to injury, the man left the room as abruptly as he had entered.

My emotions welled up inside me and I was shaking with fear and confusion. All I could think of was to get out of that building as fast as possible. Grabbing my jacket and purse I charged through the waiting room, not even looking in Steve's direction when he called out my name. As I reached the outside I started screaming four letter words between sobs and did not care who heard or saw me. Steve had followed me and now gently guided me to our car. When I calmed down enough to choke out the story, Steve was furious.

He immediately went back inside and walked into the doctor's office without knocking, where he proceeded to have a few dignified, but choice, words with him. The doctor had merely shrugged his shoulders and excused his verbal abuse of me with the fact he was so busy and had had an emergency case with one of his patients. Steve and I were thoroughly disgusted with the arrogance of so many of the doctors.

Eventually, my doctor explained to me that the term "end out" meant that the blood vessels of my eye were no longer bleeding and it was possible they never would again. He said he did not know what was causing the blurriness. I showed him my new glasses but he had no interest in them. I asked if the work I did was detrimental to my eyes. He said it could be, but he did not know for sure. After all this, I was no closer to an answer.

When I discussed my problem with Anne, she said my eyes were far more important than the job, so we agreed that I would quit working, take it easy for a while, and see if my eyes improved. I informed the teacher I was resigning and she seemed sorry to see me go. I said I had enjoyed the children, and then I left, with no regrets.

Ironically, months later, I came to the conclusion that the blurriness was actually caused by the intense strength of the magnification in my glasses. Because I constantly took them on and off all day, my eyes never had a chance to equalize or relax. If either of the doctors had bothered to look at my glasses, a lot of grief could have been spared.

Finding the special glasses did more than enrich the quality of my life. Also they had indirectly led to my confrontation with the different doctors and, because the doctors had failed me, I was learning to trust myself more and not take no for an answer when there was something I believed in. I had to accept that doctors did not always have answers, or the right answers, or my best interest in mind.

Also, the fact that I could read now put a whole new light on my employment possibilities. I wanted more responsibility than just being a teacher's aide. I told Steve I thought I could handle being a certified teacher in Special Education — after all, it was what I had trained for in college. He was behind me all the way. The newspaper he worked for was going out of business, and we decided it would be an ideal time for us to make a big move. I wanted to go to Albuquerque because I missed my family and Steve liked the idea.

I spent the summer writing up a resumé and sending out applications, thoroughly enjoying the process because I was doing the work by myself. I even flew to Albuquerque for interviews. Each major move in my life had led to something good and I anticipated that our move to New Mexico would too.

When Steve and I arrived in October, I already had a strong possibility for a job. It was as a teacher for deaf/blind, multiply handicapped children at the state institution. At the interview, I told the Director of Education that my having the personal experience of being visually handicapped would, I believed, make me a better teacher. She very much agreed with me and offered me the position, which I accepted. When she told me I would earn $1,000 a month, I could hardly believe my ears. My job as an aide had only paid $100 per month.

This was to be the most demanding job I had had so far and my confidence in meeting the challenge was high. I had one teacher assistant, six nonambulatory students, and my own classroom. The first several months were a real eye-opener for me, as I tried to adjust to the ins and outs of working for a state-run, bureaucratic organization. More often than not, one-to-one time with the kids was interrupted by meetings, tour groups, and unscheduled activities. I had mountains of paperwork, which I took home every night. The longer I was there, the more able I was to have and express an opinion about my teaching philosophy and about the way the school was run. I loved my students and cared very much about the work I did with them. When it was in their behalf, I learned to openly question or disagree with the staff, doctors, and administrators. This attitude of strong principles did not make me popular, but I felt better about myself. I was amazed at how assertive I was becoming.

My new, more aggressive attitude, which teaching was helping develop, was happening for a reason. I would soon be drawing heavily on my strength and positive thinking, along with my family support system, as I entered the most dynamic—and life-threatening—period of my life.

Chapter Eighteen

BOTH FEET ON THE GROUND

I WAS IN THE middle of my second year of teaching when a seemingly minor incident blossomed into a major crisis and redirected my attention back to my health.

Prior to this event, my body was sending out subtle messages that all was not well internally, but, par for the course, I would overlook them, put up with them, and worst of all, disassociate them from my diabetes. One was my teeth. I had had eight teeth crowned in the previous two years and each dental check-up revealed at least six new cavities. It never dawned on me then that too much sugar in my blood, as well as too much sugar in my mouth from sweets, might be harming my teeth.

Another thing was my hands. I noticed that when I cut or scraped them, they did not heal in the usual way. The scabbing process would begin, but instead of the entire scab falling away in a week or so, a tiny part of it would remain, and then thicken and deepen. If I tried to remove the scabs, small holes surrounded by darkened red skin were left. The scabs and/or holes would linger for weeks and were painful when bumped.

None of these things seemed crucial, because I generally felt healthy and energetic, which was what I always went by. My vision had not changed, I rarely had insulin reactions, and my neuropathy bothered me only when it was humid. But, I continued to overeat and never tested my urine for sugar content.

Foot trouble, of any kind, was the farthest thing from my mind. Over two years had passed since the bones in my foot dislocated, and I was accustomed to the way my foot looked. My foot was doing so well that several months before, I stopped wearing the brace, mainly because it hindered my work at school. There was no pain and it was wonderful not to limp anymore.

One morning, while getting ready for school, my right, big toe felt tingly. Steve looked at it and said there was only some slight redness. By noontime my toe was quite swollen and bright red. I decided to go see the endocrinologist who had treated me in high school, and whom I saw once in a while since moving back to Albuquerque. He thought my toe looked irritated from an inbedded splinter but when he tried to dig the splinter out, it produced only blood.

He prescribed antibiotics, told me to soak my foot in warm water, and to stay off of it as much as possible. He was leaving the next day on an extended vacation, and I was to call him when he returned if my toe was no better.

Another week brought no change. I was getting restless and felt irritated with my doctor, who had not known specifically what was wrong with my toe, but went ahead and prescribed the "catch-all" for diabetic problems—antibiotics. So, why weren't they working?

I was growing weary of traditional medicine; it had never helped any of my side effects. I read about vitamin therapy, special diets, and mental healing. Now I thought I would try fasting, in hopes of cleaning out my system of whatever might be infecting my toe. I drank liquids, but ate no food and cut back on my insulin dosage. I started eating food two days later because the swelling spread to the rest of my toes and the bottom of my foot. I continued to feel good, however, and did not think my blood sugar was being affected. What I had failed to consider was that when the body is in trauma more insulin than usual is required. I should not have tried something new while my body was under stress.

The swelling came and went from day to day, and my foot changed color from red to a mixture of red, purple, and green. On the day it was swelling, it also felt more numb. I thought of calling another doctor, but didn't want to see someone unfamiliar with my case. Steve said my foot looked like blisters were forming, so I tried puncturing the skin to see if it would drain. But it would not. I continued with the soaking and concentrating my thoughts on healing.

About ten days after I had seen my doctor, I got a fever and began having chills off and on. The lower half of my foot turned black. It looked like the skin could be peeled right off. When Steve came home from work, he took one look at my foot and said I was going to see a doctor the next day. I agreed, but reluctantly. I kept thinking that if I just waited a few more days, it would all clear up.

The doctor at the emergency room was very alarmed when he saw my foot. He said it looked like the beginning stages of gangrene, but there was nothing he could do but confer with a surgeon. Steve and I were dumbfounded, for we had no idea the condition of my foot was that severe. The doctor suggested I check into the hospital. It was likely I would need surgery.

At hearing this, my mood was a jumble of emotions. I dreaded the thought of going to the hospital again, but I also hoped that the surgery would relieve the tremendous pressure in my foot.

Steve stayed with me until I was admitted to my room and then left to pick up a few of my things. Only ten minutes elapsed when a Dr. Bryant (not his real name) rushed into my room and said that he was the surgeon on my case. He explained that he had just seen my x-rays and that my foot was in terrible shape. Gangrene had set in and he would have to put tubes in my foot to drain the infection. He spoke quietly and with earnest as if time was an important factor.

In contrast to him, a sudden wave of calm swept over me as we talked. The roller coaster that my emotions had been riding for the past two weeks came to an end. I desperately wanted my foot to heal, no matter what it took. I had a certainty within that everything would be all right, and I was free of any fear or anxiety at what the surgeon was saying to me.

I smiled at him and I must have been wearing a very relaxed expression, for he looked at me quizzically as if I did not take the matter seriously. He was unaware of all that was going through my mind and I did not elaborate.

He asked about anesthesia and I told him I was sure he did not have to put me out since I had very little feeling in my foot due to neuropathy. He hesitated, as if he wanted to trust what I said, but then decided I would have a spinal block. I could not have a general anesthesia because I had eaten lunch and vomiting had to be prevented.

Forty-five minutes later I was on the operating table in a room with low ceilings and bright lights. First, I sat on the edge of the table so that the block (medication) could be injected into my spinal column near my tailbone. It did not hurt. Within minutes I began to lose feeling from my armpits down. I tried contracting my right calf muscle, but there was absolutely no awareness of that part of my body. It was eerie to say the least.

I directed my attention to all the activity going on around me — my first time awake in an operating room. I could see various machines and five people bustling about in the small area. It was hard to distinguish between doctors, nurses, or attendants because of their identical green caps, gowns, and face masks. One put a blood pressure cup on my right arm, one put an I.V. in my other arm, and one placed a surgical cap on my head.

I was impressed at how each of them, busy at a specific task, were still being polite to one another, and friendly and reassuring to me. My comfort seemed to be of utmost importance. I was shaking uncontrollably from the fever and chills, and an alert nurse, who had already noticed, soon brought blankets that had been warmed in a dryer and put them over me. They felt wonderful and I thanked her.

Dr. Bryant entered the room and asked how I was, to which I replied, "Great!" I was experiencing such peace.

While the operation was in progress, I was unable to observe it because a draped tray was placed over my waist area, but I could hear everything that was said, and it was all connected to the surgery procedure. I trusted all whose care I was in and believed all would go well.

I decided to put into practice some of the healing techniques I had been learning and reading about. I began by creating a mental picture of my foot — the way it was supposed to look — and then of all the things I would be able to do with healthy feet: walk, run, skip, jump, climb stairs, and go barefoot in wet grass, feeling the water on my toes. I was so absorbed with my visualization that when someone spoke to me, I had to remember where I was. I was truly happy.

Surprisingly, the operation was over in 20 minutes and I was wheeled to the recovery room to wait for the anesthesia to wear off. A nurse sat beside me in a partitioned area. My jubilant mood continued and we laughed and kidded. All at once I heard my mother's voice from behind the curtain calling my name and asking how I was. I told her how I had visualized during the surgery. Mother, who had not known I was coming to the hospital, was joyful at my positive attitude and said she believed I could do what I said.

We talked back-and-forth awhile and then I spoke to Hank, Lisa, and a friend, and I had them all in gay humor. Only Steve was allowed to come behind the curtain to visit me. When he saw my carefree countenance, he too was encouraged by my mental efforts.

Two days later Dr. Bryant operated again and this time he had to remove parts of my foot — tissue and skin that were dead or too diseased from the gangrene to be saved. Afterwards he came to my room and told me that even at this point, he was not sure that all the diseased tissue was gone, and he wanted me to be aware that it was possible that I might lose my foot. The critical factor was whether or not the infection had gotten into my bone, for if it had, my foot would definitely have to be removed. He was calling in a bone specialist to have a look.

I was not upset. Even the enormity of his prognosis did not phase me, although I was admittedly shocked at what the unwrapped bandages revealed. On the top of my foot just under the toes, there was a two inch by one inch hole, about one-sixteenth of an inch deep. The exposed surface was wet, smooth, and bright red. Another opening ran between my first and second toes, to the underside where there was a gaping hole extending from the big toe to the ball of my foot. This hole was three-fourths of an inch deep and had an irregular surface. My foot was quite swollen also. I was quite in awe of it, but decided that one look was enough. A friend who was visiting one day described my foot as looking like a piranha had gotten hold of it. Her none too delicate, but accurate description made me chuckle.

The bone specialist agreed with Dr. Bryant that my foot might not make it. I, of course, did not accept his verdict and I stood firm about getting a second opinion. I was a bit surprised when Dr. Bryant readily complied with my request. After the second specialist examined my foot, he immediately declared that it would take a good six months, but my foot would definitely heal. I had almost expected his words and I felt like hugging him! Six months seemed like an exaggeration, but that didn't really matter — as far as I was concerned — my foot was saved.

I sensed that Dr. Bryant was troubled by this new prognosis and had not expected it. He told me I would have to stay in the hospital at least two weeks until the healing process was well underway. Day-by-day as he saw my foot, his doubts turned to belief and I could tell that he was sincerely pleased and amazed at my progress.

The care in this hospital was sloppy and inefficient when it came to my diabetes schedule. I knew I was not in good control because many of my blood sugar readings were high, and when I had insulin reactions, the staff doubted me and were slow about bringing me orange juice. They were often late with meals, snacks, and my insulin shots. Finally, I asked the doctor if I could have insulin and syringes with me so I could take my own shots. Although he thought it was a good idea and wrote the order, it was the nurses who insisted on double checking my syringes after I had filled them as if I had not been filling them on my own for 15 years.

As to my foot, it had to be soaked for 20 minutes four times a day in a disinfectant called Betadine® and then packed and wrapped in sterile gauze. I was frequently left alone for over an hour of soaking, while the nurses forgot to wrap my foot.

Despite the inadequacies of the staff, my foot was healing and show-ing signs of granulation — which meant the tissue was growing back. My morale was high and I was determined to surround myself with a posi-tive atmosphere. I had motivational posters hung on the walls, and when anyone referred to my foot as the "bad one" or the "sick one," I would smile and correct them by calling it my "beautiful foot."

Steve, Lisa, and my friends visited and gave me constant support. I talked on the phone with Deb a few times and she was very concerned about me. To keep me from getting bored, Mother and Hank surprised me by bringing a film projector and screen to my room and showing my favorite home movies of when Deb and I were babies and toddlers. We laughed at the cute, perfect little feet I had! Seeing them reinforced my belief and helped with my imagery.

By the time Dr. Bryant announced me ready to go home, the hole in the top of my foot was almost healed, but the one on the bottom was still quite deep. The wounds had to heal from the inside out, which meant the skin could not just be sewn together, the sides had to grow together. I could not believe that my foot could heal safely without me being in the hospital, but Dr. Bryant assured me I could take care of it fine. He ex-plained that he wanted me to soak my foot in water and scrub inside the open areas with a washcloth and Ivory soap four times a day. This would prevent a scab from forming before the tissue completed growing. This procedure would not hurt but was a little unnerving to carry out. I was to use sterile bandages, but no medications or disinfectants.

Over the next three weeks at home, I was diligent about carrying out Dr. Bryant's orders, and my foot continued to heal. However, during the fourth week my foot turned red and heated up. Steve and I were alarmed at this first hint of bad news. This time it was Dr. Bryant who was not worried and said there was probably some infection left. He pre-scribed some antibiotics and later, in his office, did some minor surgery on my foot.

Unfortunately, none of these remedies helped. My weeks of positive thoughts were slowly dissolving and tension and fear were taking over. When he next saw my foot, Dr. Bryant was gravely concerned and told me he was going to confer with an orthopedic specialist. I started crying because I understood the implications of this — the infection might be in my bone. I apologized for crying, but Dr. Bryant squeezed my hand in silent sympathy for what I was going through.

While he phoned the other doctor, I sat nervously with Steve in the waiting room. Both doctors agreed that I should immediately check back into the hospital. Dr. Bryant told us to meet him at the hospital admitting office that evening.

Steve and I were extremely upset at the thought of me going back in. When we met at the hospital that night, I told Dr. Bryant I had made an important decision — I would not be checking in then because I wanted to first see a nutritionist for a second opinion. Dr. Bryant was visibly upset, mentioning something about this doctor being a quack and that I would be wasting critical time.

His attitude made me boil with anger, and I could not restrain myself. In a composed, but firm voice I looked him straight in the eye and told him I did not see how he could degrade this other doctor when I had just run up a $5,000 bill, the infection was back with no explanation, and he expected me to go back into the hospital. What grounds did I have for trusting him or his specialist that things would go right this time? We argued back-and-forth for 15 minutes, and since I would not relent, he finally gave in, though he was clearly disappointed in my decision. I was glad for having stood up for myself.

The nutritionist said he could get me on a healthy program, but he could not do anything directly for my foot. His tests showed that I was extremely anemic and deficient in other minerals. I started on iron and other vitamins and minerals. A hospital test later confirmed the same, and I felt better for having gone to see him.

Two days later, in hopes of getting better service, I checked into another hospital that Dr. Bryant worked at. The evening after I was admitted I was sitting in bed surrounded by him and two diabetes specialists from the hospital. I was blunt and assertive, telling them how unhappy I had been with the former service, and that this time I expected to participate in all the decisions about my care. I also wanted insulin, syringes, and orange juice at my bedside at all times. For my part, I would keep a notebook of everything I did so they could keep a check on me. The doctors listened respectfully and consented to my being involved.

Dr. Bryant remained behind, after the others left, to tell me he was officially off the case but would keep informed of what was happening. We had developed a rapport and I was sorry to see him go. I thanked him for all he had done and we shook hands and said good-bye.

My relationship with the orthopedic surgeon could not have been more opposite. Dr. Smith (not his real name) came to my room later that night. He was rude, extremely negative, and had a terrible bedside manner. After hastily unwrapping my foot, he looked at it disgustedly and said he would operate to remove more tissue, but if the infection had gotten into the bone, he would amputate up to my heel and if necessary, up to my knee. He emphasized that this was the way it was done.

His "no beating around the bush" approach certainly held my attention, but I did not let it upset me. I calmly told him I understood what he was saying but that I wanted to give my foot a chance to heal. He seemed annoyed that I was not taking his words "seriously" and repeated twice that he didn't think my foot could make it.

I would have preferred Dr. Smith to be more optimistic, but actually, his negative attitude had the opposite effect on me; I was more determined than ever to save and heal my foot — for good this time.

When Dr. Smith operated, I was put completely out, because he did more extensive cutting. He said it went well, but his opinion was not changed. I needed a final surgery, but amputation was still a possibility. This man, I thought, would not be satisfied until he had cut my foot off.

The fourth surgery was done by Dr. Smith's partner, a much friendlier and optimistic person. Because he had to cut so deeply into my foot, it bled profusely and I vomited for several hours afterward. The surgeon said this was a sign that my circulation was good. This bit of encouraging news brought a smile to my weak face. My foot was so heavy with bandages, I could barely lift it off the bed. Steve teasingly called me "Big Foot."

This time around, my hospital care was much better. My blood sugar was in control and I felt good. In order to build up my strength, I requested a physical therapist, who taught me some weight lifting exercises I could do while lying in bed.

One day I was alone and listening to a Talking Book when in walked Dr. Bryant wearing a big smile on his face. He had just come from surgery and was in his green outfit, and his forehead and brown, curly hair were damp with perspiration. As he removed his glasses and wiped his face, he sat down at the foot of my bed and told me he heard how well I was doing and he wanted to tell me in person how pleased he was.

I wasn't sure what to say, but he was open and friendly and talked about things other than my health. He was rather relaxed since we were not in the doctor/patient role. More visits followed and I looked forward to them. It was the first time I had known a doctor as a person apart from his profession and I liked him very much. He asked me to stop by his office now and then to show him how my foot was doing. Not long before we had been at odds over my treatment; now we were friends.

Nearly two weeks had gone by and it was time for me to be released. I asked if it were possible to have a visiting nurse to keep an eye on my foot and to avoid so many trips to the doctor. The doctors agreed this was a good idea. What a relief to find out that these nurses would bring me all the supplies I needed and the bill would be sent directly to my insurance company.

It was now mid-October, 1979, and I set out to prove how fast my body could heal in an environment of good eating, good thinking, exercising, and faithful attention to my foot. I was extremely grateful to the Home Health Care nurses, whose services allowed me to recover at home. They treated me with respect and we learned from one another. They praised me for the active role I was taking, and they appreciated how patience and courage pays off.

Unlike before, I now had an elaborate, sterile routine to go through four times a day. Instead of a washcloth, I now used a Water Pic® to spray the Betadine against the open area of my foot. The spraying kept the tissue clean and moist and massaged it, which stimulated growth. Next, I put on sterile, disposable gloves, soaked a gauze roll in the disinfectant and slowly unrolled it while I packed it into the hole — now three inches wide, one-and-a-half inches deep, and running the entire length of the sole of my foot. It was kind of eerie to be touching the inside of my body. It was pink and wet with smooth bumps. Last of all, I wrapped my entire foot with yards of sterile, dry gauze.

Probably the most difficult part of my recovery was my relationship with Dr. Smith, who continued to be arrogant, narrow-minded, and skeptical. The main problem was that he had no interest in my diabetes — considering it the concern of another doctor — and therefore resented it when I tried to show him how controlling my diabetes and the healing of my foot all worked together. If he had had his way, I would have lain in bed for months, with no exercise, to elevate my foot, and popping antibiotics, which made me so sick I couldn't eat. He seemed to resent each step of progress my foot made. Maybe it was because I did not throw myself totally into his hands, and I had the nerve to speak up or question when I feared something was not in my best interest. I eventually ended our relationship by writing him a polite, but straight-forward letter.

Being so in charge of my recovery brought many rough times, but also did much for my inner strength and growth. I retained my positive attitude and took one day at a time, persistently doing what it took to reach my goal of walking.

Yea! I beat the odds of six months and my foot had completely healed within three months. The transformation of the wide gap rapidly narrowing had been a fascinating process to watch, and I wished I had taken color photographs of each stage.

During the past months, I had used crutches and a chair with rollers to get around on my left foot. Now, my dream of having both feet planted firmly back on the ground was near and yet so far. Over the next five months, every time I tried to walk, a blister would form on the ball of my "new" foot and then turn into an ulcer. The ulcer was a small, clean hole caused by inadequate healing due to poor circulation. I was seeing both my former endocrinologist and another surgeon, but their advice and attempts to heal the ulcer were in vain. One day this surgeon asked me if I had ever gone to a podiatrist. I said no, that I had always been told that they did not know enough about diabetes to care for diabetic feet. He said he had a podiatrist friend who was sure he could help me. That casual referral would change my life.

My first meeting with Dr. Giebel dispelled all my misconceptions about podiatrists. Not only did he test my blood sugar right there in his office, but he was also very aware that good diabetes control aided in the healing of foot problems.

He was fascinated by my foot and wanted to know all about my dislocation and the gangrene. When I described the tingly, red area that had started it all, he said it was very likely a type of fungus, like Athlete's Foot, which I could have picked up anywhere. This fungus, when treated properly (which was not with antibiotics), can be cleared up in a few days. I asked him why none of my doctors had consulted a podiatrist. His only comment was that at the time, they thought they were dealing with something they could handle.

As to my current problem, my foot was cleaned in a whirlpool of water, then Dr. Giebel sprayed it with some medication and taped it. He brought out a material called tube foam — a pliable material shaped into tubes. He cut a four inch piece so that a "sleeve" fit over my big toe and formed a cushion against the ball of my foot. He explained that because of my mishapen foot — resulting from the cutting of tendons, muscles, and tissues — weight bearing put unequal pressure across its surface. An analogy I heard later was that my foot, in trying to carry out its function, could be compared to an actor who is trying to perform a trick without using a stunt man to stand in for him. The tube foam pad allowed me to "roll with the punches" and avoid injury.

The best news was that I could walk all I wanted, that walking would actually help the healing process by massaging the affected area and increasing circulation. I could put away the crutches and wheelchair once and for all. Under Dr. Giebel's care, the ulcer was gone in a week because he knew what he was doing.

When I walked on both feet for the first time in eight months, free of any crutches, I was as excited as a child taking her first step. I felt fabulous and wanted to keep walking forever. I admired my new shoes as if they were the prettiest things in the world, when actually they were plain, gray, sturdy orthopedic shoes. Because of the swelling, my right shoe was men's size 13EEE. But it was what the shoes meant to me that made them beautiful.

I decided it was time to pay a visit to Dr. Bryant, my friend and first foot surgeon. His praise was genuine—he thought my foot looked fantastic. He confided that when he had originally seen my foot, he honestly believed I would lose it. He said he believed that it was my good attitude that was mainly responsible for my foot healing as fast and as beautifully as it did. I beamed at his words, so appreciating his positiveness and acknowledgment of my part.

My foot trauma had now been brought full circle. I had almost lost my foot — not because I have diabetes — but because I was given poor advice. I did not excuse any of the doctors who worked with me, and whether they gambled with my foot or health by not sending me to a podiatrist, I will never know for sure. The point is that I, as a patient, did not have the background to know of that option.

It was true that my poor control over the years had led to nerve damage, poor circulation and healing (also responsible for my teeth and gum problems, the ulcers in my hands, and the neuropathy) and once the doctors had made their mistake, these factors came into play along with the shoddy attention given to my diabetes from the first hospital.

The ignorance and mistakes were forgivable only because they were followed by my acquiring knowledge and insight. Once I made the effort to be healthy, and, had the proper people taking care of me, my body — despite the diabetes — did its part for a miraculous comeback.

Chapter Nineteen

AN EYE FOR AN EYE

I RETURNED to teaching while still on crutches and, despite the negative atmosphere surrounding my job when I had left six months earlier, and the fact that Dr. Smith put strict limitations on what I could do, I was delighted to be back with my students. A fellow employee told me that the new Director of Education also had diabetes, and I was interested because I had never worked with another diabetic.

When we were introduced, we spoke briefly and then I added in a friendly tone, "I understand we have something in common — diabetes." He glared at me in return and our talk abruptly ended. Obviously he was sensitive about his diabetes, so I did not mention it again.

I was back teaching about a month when several staff and children came down with a strange virus. I caught it, too, and was forced to go into the hospital for three days to get my bouncing blood sugar level back in control. No sooner did I return to work, when the director called me to his office for a private meeting with him and his assistant. Eying me cooly, the director asked, "Do you think you are going to get sick anymore because of your diabetes?"

I resented his question since half the people in our building were sick with the virus. "No," I said. "I'm not planning to."

Then he told me I had to sign a document promising I would not get sick. I thought the whole thing was ludicrous and probably illegal, but I signed the paper anyway to avoid an argument. It seemed he was trying to use my diabetes against me, as a bone of contention, maybe because he was having trouble dealing with his own diabetes. I wanted to develop a good relationship with this man, but now I was beginning to wonder.

Invariably, the subject of my health came up again, but not in a way I would have anticipated. My vision had remained unchanged for two years and I was not worried about it, but at a friend's urging I made an appointment with a retina specialist he had recommended. Perhaps there was a new technique or operation that could help my eyes.

I took half a day off work in order to see Dr. Brown (not his real name), a tall, pleasant-looking man, who was polite and straightforward with me. His announcement that I had a cataract on my left eye which needed to be removed fairly soon, came as a real surprise to me. For some reason the possibility of a cataract forming on my left eye — the one on which I relied the most — had not occurred to me.

Two choices were open to me. If the cataract was left on, my vision would decrease slowly, but if I had it taken off, there was a chance my vision would improve. I was convinced to have the operation after Dr. Brown told me that I would be out of the hospital in three days and with no bending or lifting restrictions.

Following the eye surgery, which went smoothly, I had to wear an eye patch, and getting around with only my right eye was difficult. Work at school was hard enough using crutches, but now, with an eye patch, it was a physical challenge to get through the day. Especially hard was the strain on my eyes when I did paperwork, but thanks to the help of my teacher aide, I was getting by.

One day the director informed me that my aide was forbidden to help me do paperwork because it was not in her job description. This was the last straw. I had wholeheartedly given myself to my work, but I was not going to be mentally and emotionally drained from working with this man. I resigned before the semester ended. I missed my students terribly, but within a few weeks, I was back to my relaxed, happy self.

Now I had time to concentrate on my vision, which seemed to be getting worse. I knew the operation was not guaranteed to make me see better, but why wasn't I seeing at least as good as before? Dr. Brown told me to be patient and keep taking all the eye drops he had prescribed. My patience held out for six months, then I started asking questions again.

The explanation Dr. Brown gave me was that a fibrous tissue had grown where the cataract had been, and I would need more surgery. His words were upsetting; why hadn't he indicated earlier that this was a possibility? He must have known months ago that everything was not right. Up until now I had been pleased with Dr. Brown and was confident in his judgment. But growing inside me was a gnawing sensation that he was keeping something from me.

I told Dr. Brown that I was no longer insured and that it might take a while to come up with money for the operation. He said it could be post-poned. In the ensuing months, I had trouble finding an appropriate in-surance company. Premiums for a young person with diabetes who had had as many surgeries and hospitalizations as I had had were outra-geous. I did not hold their policies against the companies, but I was get-ting scared about putting off the surgery, since now Dr. Brown was telling me that if I did not have the surgery soon, he could not guarantee what would happen.

During November and December I was very sick with pneumonia and had an incessant cough. I knew the strain of coughing was hard on my eyes. While still sick I finally received a letter telling me I was now covered by government health insurance. I immediately set a surgery date for late January, when I would hopefully be feeling stronger.

A few days before Christmas, while I was decorating our apartment, I remember leaning over the counter when suddenly part of the vision in my left eye simply vanished as if someone had turned out a light. I had so hoped to dismiss thinking about my eyes during the holidays, but appre-hensions came rushing back. Steve hurried me to Dr. Brown's office, and it was decided my surgery would be moved up to the first available date.

The day before my 29th birthday I checked into the hospital. That evening a nurse came into my room with a permission form for my signature. Ordinarily, I did not read these forms, but out of curiosity, I read this one. It said the doctor had permission to perform a vitrectomy. This was the operation I had been considered for back in Phoenix, in which the contents of the vitreous are replaced with clear fluid.

I told the nurse how surprised I was at what the form said, because Dr. Brown had told me that perhaps someday he would do a vitrectomy on me, but at present, he did not think I would benefit from it. Now I was uncertain about what was going on. I told the nurse I would not sign until I talked to Dr. Brown and found out what he had in mind.

The flustered nurse left to contact the doctor, but she returned later with a surgical nurse who said she'd be happy to explain about the sur-gery. She said that this vitrectomy was not the one I was thinking of. In case blood leaked from my eye during the operation, the surgeon may have to do a partial, small vitrectomy as a clean-up measure. This sounded logical to me, so I signed. I felt lighthearted and told the nurse I was going to maintain a positive attitude about it. Maybe if he had to do the procedure, my eyesight would improve.

The next morning I did not see Dr. Brown until after I was adminis-tered the sodium pentothal and was about to be rolled into the operating room. I was still coherent when he came over to the gurney to say hello. Thinking he had not heard about my hesitancy at signing the form, I smiled at him and said that it was fine with me if he wanted to do a vitrectomy.

But, I think he misunderstood me or thought I was delirious from the anesthesia, because the last thing I heard him say before I went unconscious was, "Don't worry. I won't do the vitrectomy."

Later that day I went home, and my eye ached and itched. Dr. Brown had me coming in to see him every two days and taking endless bottles of eyedrops, some of which cost $20 each. A brief two weeks later, he sprang more doom on me — I had developed glaucoma (an increased pressure within the eyeball) in my left eye. He added that the glaucoma was the result of my eye leaking blood during the operation.

At hearing this, my face muscles tightened and I had to fight to control the lump in my throat. "But," I said, "when I found out what you meant, I gave my consent and signed the . . ." I had not completed the sentence when he said, with stern finality in his voice, "You told me not to do the vitrectomy, so I did not. If I had, your eye would probably not have developed glaucoma."

His outright lies about the facts flabbergasted me. A chill ran through my stomach as I recalled his last words before the anesthesia took over. I said, "It was supposed to be a simple cataract operation, I don't understand . . .?"

"It's like mashed potatoes."

"What is that supposed to mean?" I snapped.

Now he sounded annoyed. "You have grown many blood vessels inside your eye and they are blocking the drainage system which prevents the excess build-up of fluid." I was too overcome to ask further questions. Dr. Brown prescribed another eyedrop to help reduce the pressure, and then he left the room.

I could not figure out what was happening to my "good" eye. On each succeeding visit, Dr. Brown became harder to communicate with. He was reluctant to answer questions and was defensive when he did. More than once I asked why this had happened to my eye, and he would just do what I had come to despise most in doctors — passing it off on my diabetes instead of explaining in detail what the reason was.

Three weeks went by and the eyedrops were not working. Dr. Brown said he would have to do laser surgery on my eye. The thought of more surgery sickened me, and I asked him if we could wait awhile because my eye hurt so much. He replied that the pressure was causing the pain and the only recourse was to stop the blood vessels from bleeding. Since I was familiar with the laser procedure, knowing it to be simple and painless, I said okay, but I was still not happy about it.

Laser surgery was now done on an out-patient basis, but I was required to check in three hours early. As I sat waiting, I tried to recapture the safe, hopeful feelings I had had seven years earlier when Dr. Johnson first did laser treatments on my eye, but I was unable to shake my nervous tension.

When I was seated on the stool in front of the laser machine, I placed my chin on the chin rest and, unlike the other times, my head was strapped in place to keep it from moving. Nothing could have prepared me for what happened next. When Dr. Brown shot the first laser beam into my eye, I cried out because the pain was searing and intense like I had been hit with a bullet. I did not expect this pain and thought maybe something was wrong. I tried to tell the doctor, but he ordered me not to talk or move my face in any way. He paused a few seconds, just long enough for the pain to subside, and then he started up again.

With each click of the machine, my eyelids tightened in agony. When I moaned, Dr. Brown would say that it was almost over and that he had to hit the critical areas. Tears were streaming down my face and I could hardly catch my breath because the head strap was so confining. Only once did he apologize for the pain, but it sounded so insincere I was not at all comforted.

Fifteen minutes later the torture was over. I was exhausted from pain and tension. A nurse unstrapped my head and I sputtered, "Why did it hurt so much? It never hurt before!" He matter-of-factly said it was because my eye was bleeding so much. How I hated him at that moment for his indifference to me, and I wanted to strike or kick him so that he too would feel pain. My eyes were but objects to him, and it seemed like he could care less about the person who owned them.

My left eye hurt continually for weeks afterward, and both eyes were sensitive to light. I kept them closed most of the time for a minimum of comfort. Unfortunately my troubles were not over. I had yet another, fourth surgery, which according to Dr. Brown, was imperative to stop the glaucoma. As usual, the prognosis was, "We'll have to wait and see."

Finally, although much too late, I went for a second opinion. This doctor agreed with everything Dr. Brown had done and I found out later they were colleagues, so who knows if it was an objective opinion.

The only good news was that the pressure in my eye was now in the high normal range. Over the next six months, the scenario was the same—Dr. Brown, being overpolite, would check my eye pressure and tell me it was fine and to continue with the drops. He seemed so satisfied with my eye pressure that I assumed this was the key to everything turning out okay, and I waited patiently for my eyes to feel better. The only diversion from pain was the concentration required to see with just my right eye.

I stopped asking questions of Dr. Brown because I received no answers. Although I did not want to continue seeing him, I was afraid to stop. He was supposedly the best in town for my type of problem and I felt trapped.

At the end of the summer my father and his family surprised me by arriving unexpectedly in Albuquerque and inviting me to drive back to Kansas City with them. I decided getting away was just the thing I needed. My vacation stretched into two months and I had a wonderful time. It was the longest I had visited my father since I was a little girl. My eye pain minimized and I was getting used to the way I saw.

During my stay someone in the family was curious about why my left eyelid was always partially closed. I had said I was not aware of it, but it was probably because I spent so much time with my eyes closed and, my left one was still quite sensitive to light.

When I saw Dr. Brown again in October, I asked if I should be doing some sort of exercises to strengthen my left eyelid muscles which had become so weak. He paused slightly and then told me that weak muscles were not the problem. My eyeball was shrinking because of the diabetes and the excess scar tissue (produced by surgery) and there was nothing I could do about it, since it is the bulk of the eyeball which keeps the eyelid from drooping. He offered no further explanation of how this happened or what the ramifications were.

My stomach sank and I felt numb. I wanted to scream and swear at him, but words would not come. Instead, I sat there staring at Dr. Brown's eyes and thinking, "Even now you don't have the guts to tell me."

He avoided my eyes and appeared very uncomfortable. In a few seconds he stood up and rushed from the room. I waited a moment to see if he might return and then got up and walked slowly out of his office, knowing I would never intentionally see this man again. The instant he had mentioned the word "shrinking," I realized that the vision I had lost would never return and that my left eye was slowly going blind. This realization gave me a feeling of sadness and loss.

As opposed to the episode with my foot where I had gained so much insight about myself and accepted it as a basic positive experience, I sensed only bitterness and regret about my eye. In retrospect, I believe that Dr. Brown knew as far back as the second surgery, when he had chosen not to do a vitrectomy, that that had been a grave misjudgment. Then, when he was unable to control the glaucoma with eyedrops, the final two surgeries were desperate attempts to make up for the mistake and save my eye. But it was too late, and too many surgeries too fast only caused me more damage and pain.

If Dr. Brown had been honest and open with me, I may have understood and had some respect for him, despite his mistake. But I had learned only contempt and mistrust and even at that, I did not know if I had the right to feel that way. For years I had made mistakes and poor judgments with my diabetes, and now, when payments were due, my reaction was shame, regret, and an overwhelming helplessness. When was it all going to end?

Chapter Twenty

IT'S NOT OVER YET

SOMETHING inside of me always believed that there had to be an end to the course of stormy episodes I had been following for 18 years. What I had persisted in was gradually destroying my body and disrupting my life, and it was not what I wanted to be doing, but it was the only existence I knew.

Even when things appeared to be turning around, change was slow and hazardous. On my way to becoming better I had a few more lessons in survival to experience.

In December 1980 I voluntarily checked into the hospital. Although it was the worst stay I have ever had, it was also an important turning point in my life. I was admitted because a minor virus prevented me from controlling my blood sugar, and thus healing at home. I ended up with pneumonia and sicker than when I had entered, and in 12 days I ran up a bill of $10,000. But it was the frustration generated by these problems that led to my making significant changes.

I told my doctor that I had to find a way to control my blood sugar on a day-to-day basis so that I would never get this sick again. Before I checked out, he sent a home teaching nurse to see me. The nurse asked if I had ever heard of "home glucose monitoring." I told her how years previously in a university hospital I was shown how to test my blood using special strips, but I had trouble reading the results and I did not like lancing my fingertip. She said she could teach me to read the strips, and as for the lancing, there was a new product to be available soon, called an Autolet, which would prick my finger for me to obtain the blood.

In the meantime, she said there was a method for obtaining blood which was less painful than jabbing my finger with a lancet. The technique seemed to be a little severe and complicated for one drop of blood, but at this point in my health, I would try anything. It involved using a sterile insulin syringe to draw blood from the veins on the back of my hands. After watching her demonstrate, I tied the tourniquet around my wrist to pump up the veins and then tried sticking the needle into a vein. I had some trouble seeing what I was doing but the nurse guided the needle right in. The procedure took less than five minutes and seemed easy enough to try for awhile.

For the next two weeks a visiting nurse came to my home to help me draw blood for my morning test, and soon I realized that my first smooth attempt had been beginner's luck. I just could not see where the blue veins were in order to puncture them at the proper angle. Also, matching the test strip's color to the color chart was harder than it had been six years before.

The test had to be taken four times a day, and Steve agreed to help me when the nurse wasn't there. He knew how vital they were and did not want me to give up, but he did not have much better luck than I did. We simply were not as experienced as the nurse at finding and controlling the veins, and we both became frustrated. My hands were black and blue and sore, and half the time, we could get no blood at all.

Luckily, the Autolet soon arrived from California. It worked perfectly! The small, black gadget was similar to a counter that is used for adding up numbers. When the button was pushed, a spring-powered lancet was driven into my finger, which I then squeezed to get the blood. The pain, when there was any, was minor. I began regularly testing and, for the first time in my life, got a true picture of just how much my blood sugar level jumped around. Diabetics try to stay in the 65 to 175 range, and I could be as low as 40 or as high as 350. As per the nurse's instructions, I took a small amount of extra insulin whenever I was high.

About one week into using the Autolet and testing without the help of the nurse, I was scheduled to have one of my surgeries for glaucoma. While in the hospital, I had to rely on the laboratory blood tests. As soon as I came home Steve and I tested my blood several times throughout the day and I stayed in the normal range, and even a little low, even though I was eating the usual amounts and did not take any extra insulin. I thought that perhaps the trauma of surgery would have raised my blood sugar, but it did not. I felt energetic. At bedtime, my test was good, between 80 and 100, so I ate my regular snack and took my customary night dosage of insulin.

When I awoke the next morning, nothing around me made any sense. My eyes were extremely blurry, or something . . . I looked down at myself and could not see or feel my body, but I did seem to have a face and maybe a head. There was an unknown force holding me down and I felt this urgency to resist the pressure and try to get up, but I could not. At the same time I seemed to be whirling through space. All around me I saw paisley designs of various colors. It was so cold. Not knowing what was happening frightened me and I wanted to feel normal more than anything. I was certain that if the real me would just hang on, I would survive and be reunited with my body. This knowledge was the only thought I had to concentrate on.

Gradually, after what seemed an eternity, the paisley shapes turned into larger, blurry, white shapes. The ghostly shapes were making sounds and it was like hearing muffled voices from behind a closed door. It was as if I were in a state of suspension in a strange "other" world — there could be no rational explanation.

I had tried yelling out when I was being restrained, but no sounds came out of me. Now I heard a voice saying, "Steve, Steve," over and over, and I realized it was my voice. The only thing I heard back were the far away mumbling sounds. Then I was aware of a comforting, warm presence near me. Sensation was returning to my left hand and I realized there was another hand holding mine.

I continued to call out Steve's name and then I heard a voice close to me saying very distinctly that everything would be all right. The voice kept repeating those words and someone squeezed my left hand. The voice and hand were familiar, but I did not know whose they were, so I kept calling out.

As time passed, the white shapes floating about me became more defined, and I began to feel normal. The body that was returning to me was very cold. Not knowing if I would be heard, I said, "I'm so cold!" Shortly a warm, heavy object was placed on top of me. Now I was conscious enough to know that it was Steve who was beside me holding my hand and reassuring me. There was also a lady who was being very kind and attentive and two men talking to one another. Moment by moment, I became more alert and started asking questions. Steve told me I was in the emergency room of the hospital. This I could not understand because my thoughts were still on the eerie "brush with death" I had just experienced. When he told me it was five o'clock, I had no idea if he meant night or day.

I was famished and the lady, identified as a nurse, brought me a bottle of 7-Up, which I finished with one gulp. There was an I.V. in my right arm and when a food tray arrived, Steve had to help me eat.

Eating made me feel better and I was coherent enough for Steve to explain what happened to me. He said he awoke in the middle of the night and heard strange noises and felt the bed rocking. I was unconscious and seizuring and, although my eyes would open at times, I would not answer when he called my name. Steve tried to get me to eat some sugar but I fought him, so he decided to call for an ambulance. Two firemen got there first followed by two paramedics. All were crowded into our small bedroom and there I was sprawled on the bed wearing nothing but socks. Steve informed the men that I was diabetic and it was possible I was having an insulin reaction. Ignoring what he said, they kept asking if I drank or smoked marijuana or used anything harder. He told them no and then stood off to the side while they tried to stop my seizuring.

Two ambulance drivers showed up and Steve repeated what he had told the others. Since the medics were having no success in bringing me around, they agreed that it must be low blood sugar and decided to put a glucose I.V. into my arm. That took several people holding me down, and this was probably the·early sensation of being restrained that I had been aware of. I fought like a wild animal, but they managed at last to tie me to a stretcher and my arm to a board.

As I was being transported from the bedroom to the ambulance, this was likely what I had sensed as whirling through the air. Steve rode with me in the ambulance for the two block trip to the hospital. In the emergency room, massive amounts of glucose were put into me and by the time I began to come around, it had been two hours since Steve discovered me unconscious.

While I was eating, a doctor entered the cubicle to tell us that when I had come in, my blood sugar reading was ten, and this was the first time he had seen a blood sugar that low. Steve and I were amazed, for we assumed a person would be dead if he got that low.

By six that morning, Steve and I were back home and eating breakfast — I was still hungry. We could hardly believe what had taken place in the last few hours. The experience had certainly superceded any insulin reaction I had ever had, and I was especially dumbfounded by my temporary vision and hearing losses. We could not figure out what had brought it all on.

Later, when I related the story to my doctor, I asked what would have happened if I had not gone to the hospital; could I have died? His answer was no, that eventually my body would have "kicked in" sugar to my bloodstream. This was news to me and I was skeptical. He advised that if it happened again, Steve should put honey or Karo syrup inside my cheek, where it could get into my system even if I could not swallow. As to why my blood sugar level had gotten so low he was not positive, but possibly there was residual anesthesia in my body from the surgery. To me, this seemed like something I should have been warned about before I left the hospital even if the possibility of this happening was remote.

In order for me to avoid another drastic episode, my doctor suggested I meet with one of the nurses from the clinic who was doing a study on home glucose monitoring. Steve and I were impressed with this nurse's knowledge of diabetes and we met several times with her. She worked with Steve on accurately comparing the color on a test strip to the colors on the color chart, and she taught me how to regulate my insulin dosage based on test results—called a "sliding scale" insulin regimen. There were formulas for figuring exactly how much extra (cover) insulin to take when my blood sugar was high.

The information she gave us made sense and getting my blood sugar in some kind of control was indeed satisfying. The only part I disliked was having to rely on someone else to read the strips. If no one was around, I could not take a test, and I did not think it was safe to be that dependent on others. When I asked my doctor about this, he did not have any alternatives.

But I was not about to give up this easily. A phone call to the pharmacy I traded with provided the answer. My inquiry was about the machine I had used six years earlier, which "read" blood glucose test results. The price had come down two-thirds, to $300. I immediately made arrangements to buy one, and a saleswoman came to my home to show me how to use the refluctance meter. When a test strip was placed in the machine, a number indicating the exact ratio of sugar to blood lit up in red on a screen. A bottle of 100 strips cost $40 and I would be taking four tests a day.

It felt like Independence Day when my new meter arrived. Now I could test and hopefully control my blood sugar on my own and avoid going to the hospital for minor illnesses. My blood sugar continued to widely fluctuate, and now I knew why all my life doctors referred to me as a "brittle" diabetic.

It was late summer by the time I got my meter and Steve had moved to Southern California. He had gone ahead to find work before I followed in early 1982, about six months away. Meanwhile I stayed part of the time with Lisa in Albuquerque and part with Grandma in Truth or Consequences. I was anxious to prove to myself and my family that testing with my meter would do great things for my life as a diabetic, never thinking that I would end up in the emergency room again for the same reason.

But end up there again I did, and over the next year, similar incidents happened with every member of my family. Each time I believed I was taking the proper measures to stay in control: testing and applying the formula. The scary thing was that even when I did not go unconscious, the plunging drops in blood sugar came on so quickly that I did not have time to treat them and had to ask for help. Once, while standing in front of a mirror, my leg began to twitch. Wondering if I might be low, I turned to go get some pop. Suddenly I collapsed on the floor and had to shout for someone to get me the pop. The leg jerking went on for ten minutes, then I was okay.

Another time, during Christmas, I was reading something to Deb and, right in the middle of a sentence my hand jerked violently and I could not hold on to the paper. Mother, Grandma, and Deb all began yelling and demanding to know if I was all right. I hated being the center of a panic situation and being asked questions. When they asked me to think or respond, I got angry or confused because my low blood sugar prevented my brain from functioning properly. Even if I knew the answer or tried to explain, the words would not flow out smoothly.

Later, I told everyone that if they suspected I was having a reaction or if I was not acting quite right, to just give me some juice or pop and order me to drink it. If they said, "Denise, I think you need this. Please drink it," with an authoritative voice, I would be more likely to do what they asked and not get defensive.

The worst reactions came on while I was sleeping. I would awake during the night sweating profusely, and then I would get very cold. Although there was pop beside my bed, I was not coherent enough to drink it. Rather, I would sit up in bed, or find myself sitting up, rocking back-and-forth or slapping my arms and legs. I always had the feeling I was losing my body and by slapping or moving it, I knew I was still there. These actions must have also helped my body release stored sugar for energy (what my doctor had referred to as "kicking in"), because slowly I would feel my body returning. How much actual time elapsed I do not know, but then, when I was sufficiently conscious, I would reach for the can of pop and drink it. I hated when this happened, but at least no one was around to panic or ask questions. Later, my blood sugar was always sky high.

Because he was the most familiar with them, Steve quickly learned to use common sense. A year after the first "bad" low, Steve again awoke during the night to find me seizuring and in a cold sweat. Since no honey was available, he decided to try and give me a Coke. I was no help and clenched my teeth tightly together, but Steve patiently forced my mouth open and fed me the liquid one drip at a time. It was an hour before I began to show signs of life, and Steve had succeeded without a big ambulance and emergency room bill.

By far the most dangerous of these events happened in the summer of 1982 after Steve and I moved to California. Steve was across the complex doing laundry and the last thing I remember doing was sitting at my desk writing. Although I took frequent walks around our neighborhood, this time I did not know how I ended up outside. I just knew that I was, and that I was moving forward. Everything around me was blurry and unfamiliar, but I still had an awareness of my body from about the waist up. At times I knew I was crawling on the ground, but had no memory of falling. Then I would be up again and weaving from one side to the other on what appeared to be a road or a field. Occasionally I saw a car or another person — they meant no more than seeing a tree or telephone pole. As with previous times I had an overwhelming urgency to get somewhere or to feel something.

A small white car pulled up beside me and I heard the pleasant, concerned voice of a girl asking if I wanted a ride. I hesitated and was about to say no, but was alert enough to know I better take help when it was offered, because I really did not know where I was. The risk was necessary, however. If the stranger had been a man, I don't know what my response would have been.

Climbing into the car I noticed a second girl in the back seat. We started driving and the girl at the wheel asked me where I lived. Despite my drunken-like behavior, I repeated my address like a robot. Also, I mumbled something about my blood sugar being low as I did not want them to think I was on drugs.

The ride was surprisingly short; I must not have been that far from home. We drove into the parking lot and I saw Steve walking toward the car. I told the driver she could let me out. I thanked them and they drove away.

Steve looked very relieved to see me. He opened the can of pop he was carrying and handed it to me, and he listened quietly while I pieced together what had happened. He told me he had discovered I was gone and knew something was not right because I had left the door wide open, and I had not taken my keys or bag of sugar cubes with me. I now saw that I was wearing shorts, and I never went out in them. My knees were scratched and bleeding. Neither of us knew the entire story.

Steve was upset, saying I was dangerous to myself if I could leave the apartment without knowing it. We had to do something to avoid these low blood sugar nightmares. When we got inside, he took out a sheet of paper and said he was going to write down everything. For the next few days he made me keep track of every move I made: when and how much I ate; when and how much insulin I took; what time I exercised. After all he had been through with me, I could not blame him for being so insistent, but the old feelings of doctor versus bad diabetic came over me. Admitting this to Steve was hard because — unlike the doctors — I knew his primary interest was in helping me. I told him I would take over the charts and be fully responsible for them. He agreed but said he wanted to be able to check them anytime if he had questions at all whether my blood sugar was low.

Keeping charts had never seemed important to me, but thanks to Steve I soon began to appreciate their value and purpose. No medical person had ever explained that the charts served more or less as a "memory guide" and "next move indicator." For years, ever since getting diabetes, I had tried remembering all the information and always thought I had an accurate memory. But, by keeping the charts so diligently I saw that often what I had thought I had done at a certain time, I had actually done earlier or later. It took time to see the advantages of charting.

For example, if I felt low (low in blood sugar), I could check the figures and see when was the last time I had eaten or taken insulin, and thus determine if I really needed extra food or sugar or if my last meal had not yet taken effect. The charts also made it clear how long it took my insulin to peak (point of strongest effect). Just because a certain type of insulin was supposed to peak in so many hours, obviously it varied from person to person and from circumstance to circumstance.

Steve and I now realized that the reason the formulas I had been given did not always work was because I was not looking at the whole picture of my diabetes and how my body responded. With slight variances in the formulas, I could adapt them to my individual needs.

I had always believed that the only reason to write it all down was to show the doctor. In fact, for years the only records ever requested by any of my doctors was a chart showing urine test results. I was not aware I could expand the documentation and use it to guide me through each situation and each day. What had seemed so apparent to doctors and nurses — or perhaps they had not comprehended a chart's potential — had gone right over my head. Instead of looking at the chart-keeping as a punishment or score card, I began to see it as a tool to help me control my diabetes independently and effectively. This lesson was a long time coming.

Chapter Twenty-One

A NEW ME

"ONE GOOD THING leads to another" was certainly proving to be true for me. As I became more experienced at testing my blood and keeping charts, I saw that these tools were definitely bettering my life. No longer was the controlling of blood sugar only an elusive theory—it had become a reality.

It is not that things always went perfectly or smoothly. They were sometimes a real uphill battle. The truth is that along with the freedom of monitoring my own blood also came new responsibility and frustration. Before I had begun testing, I was ignorant of the wide fluctuation in my blood sugar levels and therefore I did not think of them that often, unless they led to trouble. But now, with the testing, I was continuously aware of whether I was too high or too low, and I placed a constant demand on myself to be "normal."

There were days when I did everything "by the book" and still ended up with reactions or blood sugars over 300, and it could be nerve-wracking to say the least. I would go though periods of thinking that the safest course to take was to remain at home 24 hours a day where I could keep a strict schedule without interruptions, as it seemed the slightest variance in my routine would throw off my balance.

Many a time I got very down on myself for having a poor blood test reading, especially when it was high. It was like being graded at school—"pass" was a number below 170 and "fail" was a number above 170. I hated starting off my morning with a "failing" grade and I would usually feel momentary anger and guilt.

But gradually I came to see that the overall picture was more important than the intermittent, bouncing blood sugars. I had to work at remembering not to take it all so seriously; even a sense of humor helped. The Glucometer, which is the meter that evaluates my test strips, reads

"HI" for blood sugars over 399. When my first test of the day was such a reading, I would tell Steve, "Well, my meter said "HI!" to me this morning."

I think it was both the progress I was making in this area along with the wonderful influence of living in Southern California—and its emphasis on the outdoors and fitness—that led me to start dealing with some of the other problems in my life. The first challenge I faced was to lose the 15 or 20 pounds I had gained while living in Phoenix. I had been talking about losing weight for years, always with the built-in excuse that my metabolism was mixed up because of the diabetes and any weight loss would have to somehow just happen. Still under the impression that I did not eat that much, I figured that increasing my exercise was the only answer. In my confused way of thinking I thought there was only one way for me to burn fat. During each exercise session, my body would first have to burn up all the sugar in my bloodstream and then turn to stored fat for energy. But this, I feared, would bring on an insulin reaction causing me to eat extra and thus defeating the purpose of the exercising.

Steve put my irrational ideas to rest one day with a simple explanation, "Since you are now keeping your blood sugar close to normal, why don't you proceed as a person without diabetes? The basic theory behind weight loss is to burn more calories than you consume. A nondiabetic, with normal blood sugar, loses weight by putting this theory to practice and reducing his daily total of calories. You should be able to lose weight in the same way."

What he said sounded logical. I bought a book on dieting for diabetics and began to study what I ate in more detail. Many years had passed since I followed a meal planning book, and it was obvious I was now eating more fats than I needed. When counting calories, fats add up the quickest and I was getting mine in fast foods, beef, cheese, eggs, creamed soups, and salad dressing. The quantity of my diet had been less harmful than the quality.

My first remedy was to stop using salad dressing altogether and in many cases, plain yogurt was a suitable substitute. I also cut out 99 percent of the beef and switched to milk products with only 1½ to 2 percent fat. As the days went by I discovered many ways to decrease the fats I was used to eating. When cooking, I used only half of the beef, creamed soups, egg yolks, and tomato sauce (which raised my blood sugar) I had previously used. Before broiling chicken, I removed the skin and as much fat as possible. I steamed fish and used no breading or oil. Fresh fruits and vegetables were always a part of my diet, but now I increased the amount of fiber by eating more whole wheat bread, low salt and no sugar cereals made of bran.

Once I got started, it seemed so easy to be doing these simple things. By limiting fats, cutting calories was relatively painless as I could eat a little more of the other foods without feeling deprived or hungry. I concentrated on enjoying the food I was eating rather than on whether or not I would lose the pounds.

In conjunction with my new way of eating, I decided to increase my exercising from the dumbbell-lifting and short walks. I wanted to tone my body and avoid having loose skin when I hopefully lost weight. I began swimming laps 15 minutes a day in our apartment pool, which wasn't much but it left me invigorated. My clothes were fitting looser, and Steve noticed how quickly I was toning and firming up. After only three weeks, a friend commented on how slender I was looking. The fact that she had noticed took me by surprise, and it was then that I was convinced my efforts were paying off. Compliments of others are indeed reinforcing.

Not long after this a friend of mine from college, Noli, introduced me to an aerobics program I could do at home. Up until then I had only heard of aerobics classes, and exercising with a group did not appeal to me, but a recorded workout was ideal. Noli went through the routine with me a couple of times to try it out and I loved it. Her recommendation would add immensely to my physical well being.

I purchased a "Jazzercise" cassette and immediately started with the program. In the beginning I only did two or three of the exercises in one session. Every three days I would add one more exercise until I was able to complete the entire 35 minute routine nonstop. Eventually my workout would last one hour and 20 minutes. Because of the deformity in my right foot, it was necessary to adapt some of the exercises to my capabilities, such as: walking instead of running in place; high-stepping instead of jumping; and jogging on a small trampoline instead of the ground. I decided never to exercise if it was painful or uncomfortable, as I always wanted it to be a pleasurable experience. Whenever I was tired and planned to do only a few exercises, I found that those few always energized me enough to finish all of them.

It was true what I had heard but never before believed — my appetite decreased the more regularly I exercised, and I also required less insulin. The cardiovascular exercises (aerobics and swimming) in particular helped strengthen my lungs from the pneumonia damage and lowered my pulse rate.

But exercise did even more for me. The joy I learned to feel, the high of using my body in an active, healthy way with a goal in mind was a real motivator. Seeing my body change in shape and size because of what I had done gave me a feeling of power over my problems and made me like myself better. Pride in my physical appearance, in turn, encouraged me to be that much more diligent about my diet and controlling my blood sugar. It all fit together in a continually positive cycle. I became an exercise enthusiast and looked forward to it each day. Exercise is now a part of my life I would not think of giving up.

Not all the benefits of my change in lifestyle were as quickly realized, but were none the less considerable in terms of my overall health. In the next one to two years, I would be aware of such changes as fewer yeast infections, fewer cavities, healthier gums, and faster healing of cuts and scrapes without them turning into ulcers. I got fewer colds and the ones I did get were not as debilitating or as lengthy. Blemishes on my face cleared and discomfort from the neuropathy in my legs was greatly reduced. After all the abuse I had put my body through, I marveled at its continued ability to heal itself.

In a desire to expand my knowledge and attitude about diabetes, I resolved that it was time to read some books. By being exercise and health-oriented, my compulsion in eating was becoming less frequent, and my fear of finding out more facts was lessened. It had been my defensiveness and guilt concerning food which made me resent the diet part of being in control. Now I was ready to learn with an open mind.

One book I read was published 20 years previously which meant that the facts in the book had been available to me at any time in my past as a diabetic. To my surprise, I learned many new things. One fact shocked me because I had never heard anything like it before. Apparently some of the nerve damage caused from being out of control could be healed when the diabetic regained and kept in control for at least a year following the onset of the damage. None of my doctors had ever hinted at this possibility and maybe did not know of it. I was treated with drugs for my neuropathy and led to believe that it was a side effect I had to learn to live with.

For the first time, I finally understood why and how I had ended up in the hospital so many times for being out of control with high blood sugar. Insulin is a hormone the body uses to burn glucose in the bloodstream for energy. When there is not enough insulin (in my case, usually because I had not taken enough insulin to handle all the food I was eating), the body turns to stored fat which can be burned for fuel without the use of insulin. In a diabetic, however, this fat burning process produces chemicals called ketones or ketone bodies (acids) which build up in the body and can poison or even kill cells. This buildup can occur over a long period of time and the body will try to rid itself of the ketones by "spilling" them into the urine. When one type of ketone, called acetone, builds up, the body will also try to release it through the lungs, causing the breath to have a fruity odor—this was how my diabetes was originally diagnosed.

Other symptoms of this "ketosis" include nausea, stomach pain, and vomiting. Ketosis is brought on from insufficient insulin, illness, or too little exercise, and can be arrested with extra insulin and the regaining of control of the level of sugar in the blood. If not treated it can lead to ketoacidosis, which requires emergency medical care. If this, in turn, is not remedied, the nausea and vomiting will increase and are usually accompanied by heavy, deep breathing, as the body tries to release acid. The person will need immediate insulin and I.V. fluids (to prevent dehydration), or this condition can lead to coma and death. It was intellectually as well as emotionally satisfying to know the exact, scientific reasons behind the vague "out of control."

Through reading, it became clear to me that "controlled diabetes" and "uncontrolled diabetes" are two different diseases. In the first, with a few adjustments in habits and lifestyle, the diabetic will be "normal" in the sense that he can do the things normal people do and be healthy, maybe even more so, because he has learned to observe changes in his body. With the other, uncontrolled diabetes, comes the sickness, the side effects, and the misery. For too long I had been caught up in the vicious cycle of uncontrolled diabetes, not knowing that my suffering was unnecessary. What a difference it made in my attitude to learn about my disease. Knowledge and hope were replacing my long-time fear and resignation.

It was time to go for a medical check-up. After six months of dieting and exercising, I actually looked forward to a doctor's appraisal. The doctor was one I had not seen before. During the exam, she commented on how healthy and pink my feet looked compared to most of the diabetics she saw, and that my weight and blood pressure were ideal. I was proud to show her the charts I had been keeping, and this was the first time I wasn't embarrassed to show them to a doctor. She said my blood sugars looked good. When I told her it was frustrating to try and control the bouncing effect, she suggested a switch to a longer acting type of insulin (Ultralente) to help level them out. Her conclusion—my health was excellent. This did not surprise me because I had made a conscious effort at getting in shape and had attained the logical results.

The podiatrist I went to was also pleased with the way my feet looked. During one visit, he used a special machine to test the circulation in my feet, and found it to be excellent in both of them. Steve regularly checked my feet for red areas and blisters. One morning his exam revealed that my right foot was quite swollen and red from the ankle to the arch.

Because the podiatrist thought the swelling was the result of a sprain, I had to stay off my foot and avoid several of my exercises for many months. Finally, x-rays and a second opinion determined a correct diagnosis — traumatic arthritis. This meant that the swelling had not occurred from any recent injury. Rather the trouble had been building for years and was due to a disproportionate pressure on the bones in my arch, following the dislocation eight years earlier. The doctor said the swelling might continue to come and go, or stop all together, but that walking would not make it any worse.

This news saddened me when I thought of all the trauma my poor foot had been through. I had long since accepted the shape of my foot, never considering — and never told — that the bones would slowly continue to move out of place. Several measures were taken to alleviate the pressure. I had minor surgery to straighten my toes, wore an elastic band around my arch, and used orthotics (leather molded foot supports) in my shoes. Also, I took a tip from a T.V. exercise program which said that thick socks and jogging shoes should always be worn during aerobics. Before this I went barefoot, and the socks and shoes provided much comfort and support.

Paralleling the start of the foot problem, I had discomfort in my abdomen after eating. For years I had put up with minor irritation whenever I stuffed myself with food, but this had increased to continuous bloating and painful gas, even though I was now eating less. When I questioned my endocrinologist, she told me that this is a common side effect in diabetics who have neuropathy, and some found certain drugs beneficial. I did not want to become dependent on the help of drugs. After reading a book on the digestive system, I knew that the added fiber and roughage in my diet was adding to my problem, but I was not going to change what I ate. What I could do was to eat slower, to eat smaller, more frequent meals, curb carbonation, and continue exercising. When I remember to do these things, the stomach pains are far less distressful.

These interruptions with my foot and digestion made me face something I did not particularly want to face. Although I was now in the best physical condition I had been in since I was a very young girl, I still had past side effects to deal with, damage that had not developed overnight, but slowly from a pattern of doing the same destructive things over and over. Steve did not want me to feel defeated and he encouraged me to keep in mind how far I had come in one year. It would take awhile to reverse the damage or at least keep it from continuing and, in the meantime, I was doing the best I could by living healthfully a day at a time.

There was only one part of my body I remained self-conscious about because it was not cosmetically attractive, and that was my left eye. In the year-and-a-half since I had last seen an eye doctor (Dr. Brown), my eye had changed drastically, and there was no amount of keeping in control that would help it now — the vision was totally gone. The iris area was quite pink with tinges of green, and no pupil was visible. Unless someone really stared, these imperfections were concealed by my half closed eyelid and thick glasses.

Despite the tenderness and frequent itching, I did not think of my eye that much, and when I did, I tried to visualize it as healthy and beautiful. The vision had disappeared slowly and I adapted to seeing with only my right eye. At times I forgot I was seeing with just one eye, that is, until I knocked the left side of my head on a cabinet door or bumped into someone with the left side of my body because I did not see them.

At the urging of the doctor who treated my diabetes, I went to an ophthalmologist primarily to have my right eye checked. Photographs of the inside of that eye proved that no bleeding was present in the retina. Concerning my left eye, I half expected the question the doctor posed to me, "Have you ever considered getting an artificial eye?" I told him yes but I was not emotionally ready to have my eye taken out. The doctor explained that this was not necessary as there was a man in Los Angeles who could make me a "scleral shell" — a kind of large contact that would fit over my own eye and would be painted to look like my right eye. Intrigued by this "shell," I wanted to find out more and made an appointment with the man.

The man Steve and I met was O. Robert Levy, an ocularist, who is one of the best in the world at making ocular prosthetics. Mr. Levy had a witty sense of humor, making me feel relaxed and excited about the idea of getting a scleral shell, which he said I qualified for. He brought out a sample of both the shell and a regular prosthesis for us to study. They were very much alike except for the shell being slightly thinner, about one-eighth of an inch thick. They were made of a white, extremely hard plastic and had a slightly flattened, half globular shape with the cornea protruding to a rounded point. Weighing only a few ounces, they were about an inch in diameter. The circumference was round except for the straight, inner, upper edge which Levy said would lie against the bone of the nose. Adding to their authenticity were tiny, red veins painted in the white part of the eye. The body of the artificial eye was already available in different sizes, whereas the shell had to be made from a mold taken from the surface of my left eye, so it would fit comfortably.

Enthusiastically I gave Mr. Levy the go ahead to make me a scleral shell and in a couple of weeks, the painting sessions began. I came in once a week for four, 15 minute sessions; the paint had to dry 24 hours in between. I would sit in a chair facing an uncurtained window so Mr. Levy could study my right eye in natural light. He sat at a table on which were a brush and palatte of paint and the shell. First he painted the iris — mine was a blue, yellow and green mixture. The protrusion of the cornea was done in the lab and formed with various layers of opaque and transparent paint, giving the eye a three dimensional look. "Veining" of the white area and painting of the pupil were done last.

Mr. Levy and two assistants took turns painting on my shell. The two were also friendly and informative. The girl, Beverly Hoffman, loved her work and shared interesting details and stories surrounding the making of artificial eyes and those who wore them. Her most famous accomplishment was the making of the eyes for the movie creature "E.T." This news delighted me — my eye was gaining in notoriety!

The completed shell was beautiful, but unfortunately, I was unable to wear it. The problem was that I would accidently scratch my own cornea when fitting the shell in place. The pain was severe and took a week or more of healing time, in which I could not wear the shell. Finally, the ophthalmologist told me harshly, "Why don't you quit messing around with this and have your eye taken out?" Already forlorn over the unexpected trouble with the shell, his bluntness brought on a flood of tears. I was angry too and could not stand the thought of more surgery.

Mr. Levy was understanding about my disappointment and told me there was a good chance I could successfully wear a regular prosthesis, and he would make me a second one at no charge if I had my eye taken out. For two months I wrestled with the idea. I loved my eye and the valiant way in which it had served me for so many years through all the mistreatment and trauma. Even if I had not been able to see out of it for a long time, the thought of giving it up seemed so hopeless and final.

My eye continued to itch and hurt badly. I decided to at least find out about the enoculation (name of the operation). The eye doctor was very kind and responsive when I talked to him on the phone. He said it was a safe procedure, requiring only one night in the hospital. Just the inside of my eyeball would be removed, leaving the outer cover and attached muscles intact, and allowing for total movement of the artificial eye. My empty eye would be filled with plastic beads to replace the bulk and help support the prosthesis. My main concern was if my right eye could be harmed, but he said no.

I debated for awhile longer but found myself too preoccupied with the pain, so in August (1983), I resolved that my left eye had been through enough pain and it was time to let it go. My heart ached because I had not taken care of my eye and I grieved over this final step. But I knew I was doing the right thing and, I would look more attractive, too.

When Steve drove me to the hospital for the surgery I was extremely nervous. Unlike any time in my past, I was terrified of being put under the anesthesia. After my last few experiences, I was uneasy about going unconscious and placing my body in someone else's hands. Preceding the operation, I tested my blood every fifteen minutes since I could eat nothing and I did not want to drop too low. I listened to motivational tapes to help relax me and put me into a positive frame of mind.

The surgery attendants arrived with the gurney. I felt sick to my stomach as fear seized me, and I almost called the whole thing off. Steve hugged me and said everything would be all right. As always, his assurance calmed me. He was still holding my hand as I was rolled down the hall to the elevator. The anesthesia was beginning to take affect and I was beginning not to care about anything. Smiling up at Steve I said, "Say good-bye to my little eye."

Sometimes it is lucky that we cannot look into the future, for if I had had any warning of how sick I'd be following the enoculation, the decision to have it done would have been an even harder one. The next two weeks were a nightmare filled with excruciating head and eye aches, itching, and overwhelming nausea. I lost five pounds and my insulin requirements tripled. If not for the meter and test strips, there is no doubt that I would have spent those two weeks in the hospital. I think I was so sick because my body was reacting to having a part of it removed that was supposed to be there, as opposed to a tumor for example.

A month more of healing and I returned to Levy's to have my prosthesis made. In December it was ready and I was elated to wear my second beautiful eye. My two eyes moved together perfectly and looked natural. I was feeling pretty again and my self-confidence soared.

To top things off, I had a wonderful surprise four months later thanks to the foresight and concerned interest of an Albuquerque optometrist, who fit my right eye with a soft contact lens. What a free feeling to be rid of the weight of my glasses and, without the frames hindering my side vision, I would actually see better. From head to toe, I could now show off a totally new me!

Chapter Twenty-Two

CHANGING THE LABEL

A S I WENT through my metamorphic period of learning about my disease, changing and improving my body, and liking myself better, I was able to look at my own history more objectively. I, my family, and the doctors all made mistakes, which perhaps could have been avoided had there been better communication and understanding. I saw that ignorance and lack of responsibility were the main causes for my two decades of problems and frustrations. I began to develop a philosophy of how other diabetics could be treated and dealt with in a way that lessens their fears, motivates them, and, above all, gives them a choice on how they want to live.

For years I had mused over the idea of writing a book, centering around my vision impairment, but now I had an even broader theme that would encompass my entire experience with diabetes . . . What I felt and did as a child, as a teenager, and as a young woman. I knew I could relate to the fears and bewilderment of both diabetics and the significant others in their lives.

It is not my intention to tell another diabetic what he or she should or should not do with his or her life, but rather to show and reveal alternatives. It excites me to think how healthy a diabetic could be without personally experiencing the negative things that I went through. It is not necessary to suffer if the disease is seen as an opportunity and not a curse.

I have a special empathy for young or newly diagnosed diabetics, for it is in those first weeks, months, and even years that habits and attitudes are influenced and strengthened. A young diabetic could be approached in the following manner. A nurse, a doctor, or a counselor could sit privately with a child, and in an easy to understand way, explain what diabetes could do for him if it is seen as an opportunity for good things.

Don't talk about diets, but about eating healthy foods that will make him feel good all the time. Don't speak of exercise as a necessary drudgery; instead, talk about lots of play and fun. Explain to the child that the reason he became sick was because a part of his body called the pancreas had worked up until now. Tell the child, "With a broken pancreas you can do some things that will help your body. These are things which all people should do, but which most do not. Eating healthy foods, exercising, and getting regular sleep may not seem important, but they can help your body stay as healthy as it is today."

It is important to also say, "You do not *have* to do these things. No one can watch over you and tell you what to do all your life. If you choose not to do these things, there are several things which *could* happen. You may feel tired and have no energy, and you may spend lots of time being sick — perhaps in the hospital — when it would be more fun doing activities with your family and playing with your friends. It may be difficult to do all these things — eating right, exercising, testing, charting — at first, like it was to remember to brush your teeth, but in time they will become habits and easier to do. Each day you can tell yourself, 'I am helping my body stay well so I can do all the neat things in life. I choose to do these things, not because the doctors or my parents tell me to, but because I want to.' "

Group sessions for children (or any age diabetic) would allow them to meet diabetic peers who can identify with their problems and frustrations. Without relatives or medical persons present, the diabetic children or adults could come together in a sort of "Diabetic's Anonymous" to share about what they go through. They could talk about how hard it is to eat healthfully and to exercise when everyone around them is eating junk food and could care less about exercising. They could talk about the times they were embarrassed at having diabetes and why. They could express how it feels to be labeled a diabetic and how that has changed their lives. These sessions would not be educationally oriented, but opportunities for emotional and psychological support.

For some children this type of group might be the only support system needed to help them cope with diabetes. But if resistance, resentment, or peer pressure prove to be too much, a child might benefit from personal, one-to-one counseling with another diabetic who is a few years older — such as a junior high age counselor for someone in grade school. Or, a diabetic of the same age who has had diabetes for a few years could also help in this type of arrangement. This confidant serves as a role model.

If communication between a young and/or newly diagnosed diabetic and his doctors (and his educators) is open and strong from the beginning, the diabetic will be helped from feeling overpowered by his disease. It is poor to expect that any diabetic will, or should, accept generalized explanations about his disease, about what he should or should not do, or about the possible consequences of his actions. Examples of generalized statements are: "You can't do this; you have to do this; you will get sick; and, you could go blind."

These statements are inadequate because they do not deal with the "why" or "how" of individual situations. The use of them in instructing about diabetes is not only insulting to a diabetic's intelligence, but is condescending to his ability to be responsible for himself. Explanations should be in layman's terms and very specific. Also, they should be repeated over and over or in different ways until the diabetic (or parent if the diabetic is too young) can relay back to the medical person exactly what his disease is and what various behavior, good or bad, will do to his body. Merely hearing words is not the same as one being able to express or understand them himself.

It would be ideal if parents, siblings, or close friends also learned the basics of diabetes. If they learn but one thing, it would probably be best to know the symptoms and how to treat an insulin reaction and what the diabetic means when he says his blood sugar is "high" or "low." A little knowledge could replace panic in an emergency situation. It is vital that family members do not serve as watchdogs or tattletales, but give patience and support. Unfortunately, in some families, as in mine when I was young, members will not care to learn or to be involved. Whether this ignorance stems from apathy, a lack of awareness, or from fear, it cannot be an excuse for the mature diabetic, whose life is in his own hands, to take a similar attitude.

There is something I would like to suggest to diabetics, and that is, learn to be selfish when it comes to taking care of yourself. This selfishness might necessitate interrupting or leaving a group activity because you have to take a blood test or eat a snack or exercise. You are saying, "I have to be the most important one in my life because, if I get sick, I will not be able to contribute or share in others' lives. I care about my body even if others do not."

Another part of being "selfish" about your health is finding out and learning more about diabetes than doctors or nurses are willing or able to tell you. Insist on explanations you can understand and be sure to ask lots of questions. Often a pharmacist will take the time to explain what a drug is being prescribed for or to share his knowledge about a certain subject when a doctor will not. Reading books, getting second opinions, and observing your own body are all ways of learning more.

Knowledge is empowering. The important thing is that you are the one who has to live with the results, so you should be the one to make final decisions and make them carefully. If you make a mistake, do not condemn yourself or feel guilty. Just observe what can be done differently the next time and proceed from there. Keep in mind that there is a physical, a mental, and an emotional side to diabetes and let your body, your mind, and your feelings work in harmony for a better you.

One of the most important things I have learned from having a chronic disease and visual impairment is that accepting a thing and taking responsibility for it are two different choices. For years I was an expert at acceptance — I accepted that I got sick often, I accepted that I would have side effects from diabetes, I accepted that eating and guilt go hand in hand, I accepted ignorance and lack of communication, and, I accepted that others' opinions and advice were always right or better than my own.

But the trouble with acceptance is that it infers passivity. Others admired me for my "good" attitude and yet, my acceptance was accomplishing nothing but inspiration for others. We each have our own problems, frustrations, and mountains to climb. It doesn't matter what kind of problems they are: physical, mental, emotional, financial. They all have the potential to turn our lives around for the good. They create a desire, a gap, or a loss in our lives that we can choose to fill or not to fill. It is only when acceptance moves and inspires us to act, is it meaningful at all. Inevitably, it is not so much how we feel about it but how we deal with our individual situations that is important, for that is how we grow — going from one decision to another and criticizing, observing and appraising our results as we move forward.

For too long I let a disease and its side effects speak for me. Because I believed I deserved the consequences of my shameful actions, it was hard to see diabetes as more than just my fate in life. Thankfully, now my entire perspective has changed, and I am able to see my unique "differences" as means to an end. They are a springboard I am using to bring me closer to what I want and all that I will accomplish.

How did this change come about? It is interesting that the change did not occur as a result of any of the negative areas of my life. It did not come from people always telling me that I should take care of myself; it did not stem from my feelings of guilt; and it did not come because life decided I had "suffered long enough"—I could have kept on going the way I was. I believe that what happened was that I became self-motivated, which is the most enduring and powerful motivation of all. There are several factors which stimulated this inner inspiration. For one I began to acquire knowledge through reading, testing and observing. The second was my change in habits—eating right, exercising, charting—the results of which inspired and reinforced me to continue these habits. Another factor was that I regularly listened to motivational tapes and, for the first time in my life, became goal-oriented. And lastly, I voluntarily began to be responsible for my health, not all at once, but little by little, finding that it made all the difference when it was my choice.

I am changing my label of DIABETIC: always sick, always something wrong; to DIABETIC: always healthy, always getting better. I have changed the way I see myself, and hopefully, others will also. I no longer want to be associated with poor health, handicaps, or hospitals. I don't want people to feel uncomfortable when they find out I have a vision impairment, or to panic when I have an insulin reaction. I don't want people's first questions to be, "How are you feeling?" or "Are you all right?" and, I don't want others to concentrate on what is wrong with me, but rather what is great with me.

In deciding to be healthy, I have placed a bigger demand on my mind, my body and my will. I still go through frustration and uncertainty, but gradually I am discovering that it is a challenging experience to have diabetes, because the outcome of my disease is mostly determined by what I do from day-to-day, and my self reliance is continually strengthened and broadened. I am living in the best possible time. The 1980's is the Decade for the Diabetic. Eating good and physical fitness are in. In order to live successfully with diabetes, I must make a moment-to-moment commitment to do what I have found works best for me, and a lifetime commitment to health and happiness.

Appendix

PAYING THE PRICE

ALMOST TWO DECADES of mismanaging my diabetes brought a high price not only in health, but in time and money to myself and to members of my family. This in turn brought stress and resentment on their part, and guilt and frustration on mine. Especially as my eyes and feet became more affected, my inability to drive myself to doctors' appointments and/or to drug stores for prescriptions and supplies forced me to rely heavily on others, in most cases my family.

Approximately 180 hours of driving has been spent taking me over 5,200 miles to be seen by doctors, with an additional 475 hours of waiting once in the offices of these doctors.

In terms of money, a conservative estimate of what had been paid out by me, my family, and various insurance companies over the past 24 years is $73,400. A more amazing fact is that three-fourths of this cost was unnecessary and could have been avoided had I taken responsibility for my health from the onset of the disease.

The cost of the basic necessities for the healthy control of diabetes (insulin, syringes, testing materials, and medical check-ups) in itself has not been a small amount. These costs have risen steadily from $250 per year in 1963 to $1,500 per year in 1986. In addition to several isolated incidences of hypoglycemia that required emergency room care, and of acidosis and ketoacidosis which required hospitalization, the complications involving my eyes, feet, and nerves have led to a succession of problems requiring medical attention.

With all my diabetes related costs taken together, an average of $3,060 has been paid out annually over the past 24 years. Because of the complications (eyes, feet, nerves), it will be a long time before my only costs will be for basic necessities. Putting all these figures down on paper makes me painfully aware of just how much of my life has been given over to poor health and its consequences. Below are some of the statistics of my case as of December, 1986:

MISCELLANEOUS

Self-administered insulin shots	26,995
Self-administered blood tests	10,950
Hospitalizations	18
Days in hospital	108
Surgeries	16
Number of doctors treated by	58
Hours in doctors' offices/waiting rooms	475
Hours in transport to doctor's offices, hospitals, and pharmacies	180
Miles driven to above places	5,200
Bottles of alcohol used	123
Bottles of insulin used	285
Bags of cottonballs used	60
Bottles of eyedrops	36

COSTS

Hospitalizations	$50,000
Office visits/surgeons' fees	14,200
Syringes	1,560
Insulin	1,200
Blood testing materials	3,780
Urine testing supplies	200
Cotton	35
Rubbing alcohol	60
Prescriptions	600
Blood glucose meters	530
Leg brace, orthopedic shoes	435
Ocular prosthesis (artificial eye)	800
Total	$73,400
Average yearly total	$3,060